MODELING
AND
ROLE-MODELING
A Theory and Paradigm
for Nursing

MODELING AND ROLE-MODELING
A Theory and Paradigm for Nursing

Helen Cook Erickson, R.N., M.S.
Evelyn Malcolm Tomlin, R.N., M.S.
Mary Ann Price Swain, Ph.D.
University of Michigan, Ann Arbor

PRENTICE-HALL, INC., Englewood Cliffs, N.J. 07632

Library of Congress Cataloging in Publication Data

Erickson, Helen Cook, (date)
    Modeling and role-modeling.

    Bibliography: p.
    Includes index.
    1. Nursing—Philosophy.   2. Values—Study and
teaching.   I. Tomlin, Evelyn Malcolm, (date)
II. Swain, Mary Ann Price. (date)   III. Title.
[DNLM: 1. Nursing.   2. Nurse-patient relations.
3. Role—Nursing texts.   WY 87 E68m]
RT84.5.E74   1983   610.73   82-13286
ISBN 0-13-586198-5
ISBN 0-13-586180-2 (pbk.)

Copyright assigned February 18, 1988, by Appleton and Lange to:
Helen Cook Erickson, Evelyn Malcolm Tomlin, and Mary Ann
Price Swain

Editorial production supervision: Karen J. Clemments
Interior design: Karen J. Clemments and Maureen Olsen
Logo design: Raymond N. Tomlin
Cover design: Diane Saxe
Cover photograph: William N. Tomlin
Manufacturing buyer: John Hall

First printing 1983 by Prentice-Hill, Inc.
Second printing 1988 by The R. L. Bryan Co., Columbia, S.C.
Third printing 1990 by The R. L. Bryan Co., Columbia, S.C.
Fifth printing 1997 by The R. L. Bryan Co., Columbia, S.C.
Sixth printing 1999 by The R. L. Bryan Co., Columbia, S.C.
Seventh printing 2002 by The R. L. Bryan Co., Columbia, S.C.

Sponsored by The Society for the Advancement of Modeling and
Role-Modeling

Distributed by EST Company
        7306 Anaqua Drive, Austin, TX 78750

ISBN 0-13-586198-5
ISBN 0-13-586180-2 {PBK.}

Contents

Foreword

I feel deeply honored to be writing the foreword for this book, as my close association with the authors has provided me with my most meaningful experiences in the development of my nursing practice. Each author, in her own unique way, has stimulated me to become the best nurse I could possibly be, while collectively they have been a continual inspiration.

I first became associated with Mary Ann Swain during my early efforts with nursing research. I remember so clearly the number of times my research partner and I sat in her office worrying that our data did not demonstrate the significant differences we had expected related to our specific nursing interventions. Yet Mary Ann kept saying, "But look what you do have. Look at the number of times patients said (on the questionnaire) that the nurse was the most helpful factor in their hospital experience. What do you suppose that means?" she would ask. "What were you doing that was helpful? Why was it meaningful?"

We certainly did not know then. The health teaching and pain medications we had instituted were not mentioned as helpful. But Mary Ann continued to ask. Over the years she has listened closely to all my efforts to understand my practice, and has the unique ability of finding and developing the central themes in what I have said.

Moreover, Mary Ann has provided the environment, both the physical space and the milieu, to help me and others carry out nursing research. She has provided the opportunity, as well as the research knowledge and support to help us develop and understand our nursing practice.

Helen Erickson's very special contribution to this volume, as well as to helping me with my own practice, is her extensive knowledge of great teachers and scholars such as Abraham Maslow, Erik Erikson, and Milton Erickson, as well as the others whose work appears here. More importantly, however, she has taken their work, added nursing theory, synthesized it all with a nursing perspective, and demonstrated how the resulting overall theory supports an effective paradigm (or design) to use in nursing practice.

Helen has explained many times to me the ideas and concepts presented by these scholars, and related the theory and paradigm that she and her colleague authors have developed until I came to understand. Everything Helen has said over the years has been so clear, so practical, that I am often surprised to find myself saying to her such things as, "Can we go over the story of Sue again? Why was it right for the nurses to let her be dependent on them for care?" Each time I listened, I understood more and gained new insights. Although I don't intend to stop asking and discussing, I am glad to have this volume finally available to me for as much rereading as I like.

Evelyn Tomlin and her nursing practice are a clear validation that the theory and paradigm presented in this book work, not only most of the time, but beyond my highest expectations. Evelyn has been my role model, mentor, colleague, and friend. She has often been my nurse, and sometimes even my client.

Sharing an office for the past five years has afforded us many opportunities for meaningful discussions during which we have articulated and refined our ideas about nursing. It has been Evelyn's strong practice component with example after example of clients' positive response to her nursing care that finally helped me internalize these concepts and apply them to both my practice and my teaching.

My own growth in nursing related to this theory and paradigm can be demonstrated in three clinical experiences which I would like to share with the reader. I was asked one day to provide diabetic education to Greg, a 21-year-old man whose chart described him as "hostile and aggressive." I soon discovered that he was certainly very bitter, and also that he knew a great deal about diabetes and did not need instruction. The clinic nurse had thought that more education would help him manage his insulin reactions and thus he would be able to hold a job. The doctors believed he was using his illness as an excuse to stay on welfare.

Greg's bitter attitude softened as he talked to me. He realized that I cared about him, even though he also knew I couldn't help him. I honestly tried, but I was at a loss. I even wrote a paper about this man later, to try to gain insight, but learned little. Within a few weeks, I heard that he had been committed to a state hospital.

Edith was a 50-year-old woman with vulvectomy surgery, who was described by the nursing staff as "unreasonable, manipulative, and a malingerer." She refused to participate in her care, ate little, and would not get out of bed. One nurse tried to do some contracting with her, while another tried to have the doctors provide parenteral nutrition. Most of the nurses, however, were furious with her, believing she was trying to manipulate them. I kept saying that she was really ill and simply could not do what was asked of her.

When Edith developed septicemia and died, one nurse said, "Well, you were right. She was ill." But I was puzzled. The septicemia had not been present at the start of her postoperative course. Physiologically, she had been in fine condition, which was why everyone insisted that she do her own care. I had been right, but I didn't know why. I did not understand why we failed some of our patients so utterly. I knew that persons often responded well to my approach, recognizing that I cared about them. But it was not enough, and the good feelings they had for a little while did not last.

The answers came gradually over the years as I worked with Mary Ann, Helen, and Evelyn. Thus I share my third example. Karen was a young woman recovering from surgery. She had struggled to cope with a disease, surgery, and family concerns all at once. She was angry a good part of the time and often refused to speak to us. Since I had admitted her and performed much of her postoperative care, we did have some rapport.

One morning, I was greeted by her physician who said, "Well, you'll have your hands full with Karen today. She's refusing to cough, and has announced she won't get out of bed. You've *got* to make her understand that if she doesn't do as she's told, the result will be pneumonia." He was obviously exasperated. I went to Karen. She turned away from me with lips set and arms folded tightly across her chest, refusing to acknowledge my greeting. I said, "I think you are unhappy, Karen. Can we talk about it?" She was quiet for another moment and then, still without looking at me, blurted out, "I'm not getting out of bed and nothing you can say will make me!" I replied that she was certainly right about that, and I was not going to try to make her get up. However, I told her that I was puzzled, as she had been walking all around and feeling good just yesterday. Very gently I touched her arm and she didn't pull away. Gradually she began to cry, saying she hated this place and just wanted to go home. She missed her family so much.

Karen, of course, had been well instructed on the necessities of postoperative care and its goal of discharge as soon as possible. She had even indicated, the day before, that she knew that the frequent ambulation was making her stronger. I did not know what in particular had caused her current distress, but I was no longer perplexed by this kind of response. Her posture was relaxing, so I took her hand, and said: "I don't wonder you're tired of this place, and it is lonely when your family can't visit very often. Besides that, some days after surgery are just rough. You're entitled to feel rotten! After all, your body has been through a lot. Why don't I let you rest for a while, say a half hour, and then we'll start planning how to get you home faster."

When I returned, Karen was up and making her bed. She smiled as she sat down, and let me finish the bed. "I don't know why I behaved that way. It was stupid. After you left I told myself to get moving or I never would be strong enough to go home."

Later that morning I told the physician that Karen was fine and doing all her care. He was amazed, asking me what in the world I had said to her. I replied that, since she considered me trustworthy, when I pointed out some of her strengths and my positive expectations for her, she believed me. He looked puzzled. After all, he had been trustworthy also. But then he shrugged and said that it probably didn't matter as long as she was back on track.

But it does matter. It matters terribly. Most nurses can share with me the knowledge that an attitude like Karen's that morning can become a major problem, or even a disaster. The words and touch I used were planned from a nursing framework. I helped her remember that she was stronger than she thought at the moment, but that it was okay to have a brief relapse. I indicated that she was going to do well and that together we could plan ways to achieve her goal of leaving the hospital more quickly. Her self-care abilities came forward, and no mention of pneumonia or more instruction was ever made.

The principles suggested in the care of Karen and a great deal more are described in this volume. And so I invite the readers to join me in an exciting nursing adventure as we read and reread this book. It is the book that nurses have been waiting for. Read it and become!

Mary Hunter, R.N., M.S.

Assistant Professor of Nursing
School of Nursing
The University of Michigan

Clinical Nurse Specialist
University of Michigan Hospitals

Preface

Wise and effective nursing practice stems from two basic requisites:
(1) acquiring scientific habits of thought using existing knowledge
about healthy functioning and (2) developing clinical sensitivities
and expertise so that nurses can humanely and knowledgeably intervene in health-related situations. We want, in this book, to call
attention to both and to indicate how nursing synthesizes philosophical viewpoints, existing scientific theories, clinical practice,
and research.

We begin with a brief consideration of the current sociopoliti-
cal context of health care and the role that silence about the nature
of nursing may play in that context. We cite historical precursors
for holistic nursing and the importance of emerging research in understanding the scope and potential impact of the profession. As the
foundation for our theory and paradigm, we offer a definition of
nursing that arises from our philosophical assumptions about the
nature of humanity and the role of the nurse.

Thereafter, we unfold the theory and the paradigm in the abstract and in the concrete. Using the *client's model of the world* as a
base for intervention is central to our work. Our consistent advocacy
of this point gives this work a focus not previously developed in the
nursing literature.

We have purposefully written in a direct, informal style because we do not wish to obscure important realities. We believe this work merits serious consideration, from the novice practitioner to the most experienced clinician, from the beginning student to the most rigorous scholar. We propose our conceptual formulations as alternatives to those of other nurse theorists and, since we provide detailed information on nursing interventions within our paradigm, we suggest that our work is more immediately applicable in clinical practice.

Theories are evaluated by the uses to which they can be put. We suggest that this theory and paradigm is useful to beginning students and practitioners as it provides a systematic framework within which to collect and synthesize data in order to plan effective interventions. In addition, discussions with more experienced colleagues lead us to believe that we have articulated clearly what they have experienced intuitively. Finding ways to talk about their practice, such as we give here, assists them by providing a rationalized conception to guide their practice when they encounter clients whose behavior is initially difficult to understand. A theory is also useful if it provides a framework for both expansion and elaboration of knowledge. There is much we do not know about holistic health. From our own experience we know that this theory leads to inquiry, both inductive and deductive. Using this theory, clinicians and academicians can enhance our knowledge base about how nurses facilitate the promotion and maintenance of clients' health.

We wish to acknowledge the many people who have influenced our thinking and provided support for our thoughts. We pay special tribute to our families who have provided constant reinforcement and insights; our colleagues and students who provide support, stimulate our thinking, and particularly have made us sharpen our concepts by their excellent questions; and our clients who have directed our thinking by modeling their worlds for us.

Finally, we wish to acknowledge two individuals who have served as primary mentors. The first is a faculty member who taught her students to "Look first at the person's face, then body, and finally, the equipment required to care for him. Never, never look first at the equipment, for if you do, you might well miss the person—what he or she is doing and saying is far more important than what the equipment is doing." This mentor taught us that nursing requires that we focus our attention on the person receiving our care, not on the disease or sickness.

The second person whom we wish to recognize as having molded and directed our thinking is Milton H. Erickson, M.D. When asked what was the most important thing that a nurse could do to help people, he frequently responded with "model their world." Through years of close association and repeated teachings we came to appreciate at ever-deepening levels what he meant.

We have been able to develop our ideas and study them due to the support received by the federal government. Earlier our work was supported by a grant "Influencing Compliance among Hypertensives" from the National Heart, Lung and Blood Institute (HL-17045). More recently the Division of Nursing awarded us the grant, "Health Promotion Among Diabetics: Comparing Nursing Systems" (NU-00658).

H. C. E.
E. M. T.
M. A. P. S.

Ann Arbor, Mich.

Introduction

We want to present our ideas and convey our excitement about a nursing practice theory and paradigm that we have developed over several years. It is the natural outcome of combining clinical experience, extensive readings, many hours of rumination, and clinical research. We think it is practical in every possible nursing situation because it evolved from our respective practices that have spanned a range of ages, health and illness states, and practice settings. Our comfort in presenting our model at this time stems from our repeated successes while testing it in the real world. From these varied experiences, we have derived a useful definition of nursing.

Our definition of nursing assumes the "wholeness" of human beings. The concept of wholeness implies that a person is a unit of integrated subsystems. Within our paradigm, these subsystems are the biophysical, psychological, cognitive, and social aspects of the whole person. We believe that the nature of nursing requires that nurses be continuously mindful of the interaction of these subsystems. When nurses give clients the benefit of their awareness of these relationships and consistently exercise their special expertise in giving integrated and integrative care, people benefit remarkably.

How we deliver integrated, or holistic, care will be illustrated in the pages that follow. Our clients have confirmed that such care is integrative for them by saying it has helped them to "pull things together" for themselves.

The role of the nurse, then, is to *nurture* biophysical, psychosocial, spiritual beings. When health care consumers receive such professional nursing care, they gain a perspective on how to take better care of themselves to attain a state of health that is optimally satisfying to them. They learn more about the everchanging relationships among their own subsystems. As they are assisted to make choices that help them attain a satisfying health state, they are freed from the energy-draining consequences of coping ineffectively with real or perceived stressors of everyday life. This means, among other things, that unmet psychosocial or spiritual needs will not find expression in disease. Conversely, physical ailments will not result in tragic and avoidable depletion of psychological, social, and cognitive resources.

Nurses will recognize some very familiar ground. We have integrated concepts that you have probably used, although perhaps less systematically, over the days and years of your own practice. We synthesized these concepts in such a way as to set forth:

1. *A philosophy about nursing* that describes nursing from our perspective—what it is and how it differs from, and collaborates with, other helping professions; what nursing does for society that other helping professionals are not educationally prepared to do; and

2. *A theory and paradigm for the practice of nursing* that can guide the thoughts, decisions, and actions of nurses in every nursing situation, however particular and individualized each may be.

In Part I we introduce our view of why nurses need individually to take the time and effort necessary to develop, explain, and articulate their own personal concepts related to nursing—to themselves, to lay people, and to other health professionals. In Part II we present our philosophy and definition of nursing, the theory bases we use, our theoretical formulations, and our paradigm for the practice of nursing. In Part III we put it all together for application in nursing practice. Part IV contains answers to the questions we most commonly hear from nurses as they practice or consider practicing within our framework. Finally, there is a glossary at the back of the book to help you understand our intent in using various terms throughout the book.

We present our paradigm in full awareness of the difficulty that goes with taking an integrated system and sequentially discussing its varied elements as separate components. Sometimes we anticipate concepts, and at other times we circle back to repeat them. Whenever a dynamic process goes into print, it tends to become frozen. Packaging something necessarily involves choosing what to include and excluding much else. When you have read the entire volume, we hope a vitalized reintegration will occur for you as you apply these concepts to your personal practice.

We developed our paradigm by synthesizing the work of well-known theorists, including Erik Erikson, Abraham Maslow, Hans Selye, George Engel, and Jean Piaget. It may seem presumptuous of us to compress the detailed work of these profoundly thoughtful investigators into a few paragraphs or pages. We therefore recommend their original writings and hope the brief reviews we give will send you back to these classic works. May your renewed interest and eagerness enable you to draw from them the fine detail that can enhance your ongoing personal and professional growth.

This volume is written for nurses representing all aspects of our profession. We realize that some of you will be more interested in the conceptualizations presented and that others will want concrete information about application. Some of you will be more interested in whether your philosophy is congruent with ours and others will be concerned with whether or not the concepts are researchable. With this in mind, we encourage you first to skim this book and then return to those sections of particular interest to you for in–depth study. We realize that some sections will require repeated reading for some of you. Others will not. We believe our ideas can be studied scientifically and can help nurse practitioners raise questions and seek answers related to the science of nursing. These questions can be raised in episodic and distributive practice situations, in regard to individual and group care, at every age and stage of life.

Above all, we want this book to help practicing nurses—students and graduates alike. We hope you will find it easy reading, and that as you reread it in the midst of your continuing practice, you will find its applications and implications occurring at ever-deepening levels. We hope, too, that you will find our ideas stimulating, challenging, and energizing.

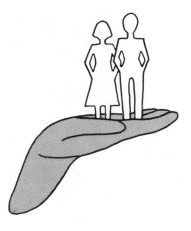

I

HISTORICAL PERSPECTIVES AND FOUNDATIONS

Historical factors influence the practice of nursing. They impact on our ability to control our profession in the total sense of the word, and they influence our interpretations of nursing. Frequently, nurses attempting to pull nursing up by the bootstraps reject their inheritance. They argue that their past placed them in subservient, male-dominated roles that are no longer useful. As a result, the positive components of the past are also frequently spurned or ignored. Nurses need to consider all aspects of our past, to identify those that work for us and those that work against us as we build nursing for the future.

In Part I we briefly assess some of these issues. We present some perspectives on historical barriers in Chapter 1 and historical assets in Chapter 2. Our goal is to encourage you to further build and articulate your own philosophy with consideration for where nursing has been and where nursing might go.

1

Why Explain Nursing?

OVERVIEW

Nursing differs from other health professions, particularly its historical partner, medicine. We give reasons why nurses unitedly need to identify differences. We describe some advantages gained when individual nurses who practice from a theoretical paradigm develop their ability to articulate nursing goals effectively.

Numerous stereotypes about nursing and three varied conceptions of the nurse–doctor–consumer triad affect our progress as a developing profession. We identify some reasons for the persistence of the former and present our concept of the differences between the terms *patient* and *client* in relation to the triad. We conclude with some practical, interprofessional, and societal implications of investing ourselves in efforts toward a full professional identity.

SILENCE OR DECLARATION: CONTRASTING EFFECTS

Distinct differences exist among nursing, medicine, and other health professions. The failure to clarify those differences and to specify the nature of nursing leaves both care givers and care receivers in jeopardy. Nurses lose control over the practice of nursing and clients receive fragmented, dehumanized services.

Many nurses practice in hospitals, schools, public health departments, industries, and health maintenance organizations. When these nurses do not unitedly declare the nature and domain of nursing practice, their institutional administrators discount the critical importance of providing holistic nursing care. Instead, administrators support care that addresses one or more of a whole person's subsystems but does not take into account the relationships among them. They expect nurses to provide sickness care designated as medical nursing, psychiatric nursing, surgical nursing (or other types of specialty care) rather than holistic health care.

These administrators frequently place constraints on nurses. They invoke rules and policies because "that's the way it's always been done." They establish nurse–client ratios without consulting expert nurses about the actual nursing care needs of care recipients; they assign workloads that do not allow the nurse time for holistic care. When forced to comply with their demands, nurses sense that they have little control over their practice. They frequently become discouraged and apathetic. Some leave the profession. Others continue, but see nursing as nothing more than a job.

We believe that personal and professional rewards proliferate when nurses take the time and effort to identify nursing goals and to design interventions based on a theoretical paradigm developed specifically for the practice of nursing. The body of specialized nursing knowledge grows and provides a base for us as we make professional judgments. We validate our effectiveness and assure the quality of our care. We become accountable *first* to the persons we serve—our clients—rather than to administrators or physicians. We gain the potential to strengthen our currently weak impact on the structures of our society that govern the delivery of health care in general, and nursing care in particular. Nurses learn how to give and receive support from one another, rather than from physician colleagues; we develop a sense of joy in nursing. If we hope to gain and maintain control over our profession and experience these multiple rewards, we must learn to explain and articulate nursing, to describe it to our colleagues, consumers, and other professionals. We believe that the quality of nursing care that we want for ourselves, our loved ones, and our clients will be realized when we are clear about our own profession—and not any sooner.

At least two major factors affect our progress. These factors are the common nursing stereotypes and the varying conceptions of the nurse–doctor–consumer triad. These will be briefly discussed below. We will not be inclusive in our discussion. Instead, we hope to raise the level of awareness of some of our readers. We assume that you have considered these issues to some extent and can add other factors that impact on our current status.

COMMON NURSING STEREOTYPES

Across time, the roles played by the various health professionals have evolved based on the needs of society. As health care has changed, new health care vocations have emerged. Misunderstandings and stereotypes have grown in the public's mind about what nursing is and what nurses do. These misconceptions flourish for historical, cultural, social, economic, and political reasons. Look with us briefly at some familiar stereotypes.

"You should have been a doctor." People often ask bright, dedicated nurses why they "stopped at nursing" and didn't "go on" or "go all the way" to medicine. Such questions suggest that many lay people (and some health professionals, too) think that nursing is somehow subordinate to medicine, that our profession is potentially a stepping-stone to a medical career, or that it is fundamentally concerned with assisting the medical profession to accomplish its important tasks for society. They overlook or misunderstand the degree of intelligence, skill, and educational preparation required of nurses to achieve their fundamental goal of nurturing persons to use their strengths to achieve optimum health. They do not distinguish the complementary health focus of nursing practice from the disease and disorder orientation of medical practice.

"He certainly trains his nurses well." Most lay people, especially those who have never received nursing care, think of nurses primarily as the doctor's helper or apprentice. A common belief is that nurses work predominantly for the doctor to take care of the sick. In fact, nurses are primarily person-helpers rather than doctor-help-

ers. Their goal is to help people with their health needs, not to care for their sickness. Such care is needed and can be provided whether or not a physician's services are simultaneously engaged. Most nurses work with people who are not confined to bed but who are up and about. Yet many people still believe that a good nurse was "well trained" by a physician. Doctors do not "train" or educate nurses. Nurses practice from a nursing framework rather than from a medical framework. Nurses are legally responsible for practicing within the parameters of a nursing practice act, not a medical practice act.

"I'm going to tell the doctor how good you are." "I've a mind to report her to the doctor."   The persistence of the notion that nurses are accountable to physicians has some relationship to the fact that ours is an emerging profession—a predominantly female one—in a male-oriented society. The male-dominated physician group earned much power and well–deserved prestige through medicine's historical evolution. That status leads many people, especially lay people, into thinking that physicians are naturally "in charge" and should therefore monitor and control nursing practice. Nursing's contribution to client welfare is too important to surrender to the direction of those whose education and expertise necessarily concentrate on different phenomena. If any hierarchy of authority is desirable, the consumer might best be perceived and encouraged to be "in charge" as the one person to whom professional helpers are all equally accountable.

"Love a nurse." "Get well quick." "Flirt with the nurses." "They've got cute nurses." "Nurses call the shots."   Finally, the mass media of our culture, especially television, create and perpetuate unflattering caricatures of nurses as not-too-bright, oversexed, ineffective, and frequently slapstick props for medical scenarios. Female nurses, wearing traditional uniforms and bearing ever-present clipboards, simply "stand by." When nurses *are* shown interacting with patients, the nurses are often portrayed as diffident, autocratic, or sadistic controllers who verbally or physically stop patients from doing something they want. What a pity that unaware viewers rarely see nurses giving even a hint of the care that real-life persons value from nurses: the facilitating, comforting, protecting, motivating, informing functions that are indispensable to persons under stress.

We have presented just a few of the common stereotypes of today inherited from various sources. We encourage you to add your own to our list. Below we briefly address why such stereotypes persist. We assume you will add to our thoughts here as well as above. We address these from three perspectives: the physicians, the consumers, and the nurses.

WHY STEREOTYPES PERSIST

The Physicians

Some physicians certainly play a role in reinforcing stereotypes. While individual physicians may not consciously adopt superior stances, many do not readily treat nurses as professional equals who have different and complementary skills. Although physicians acquire nursing knowledge over time (and often use it serendipitously in their practices, just as nurses acquire medical knowledge and use that knowledge while delivering nursing care), most physicians have not yet learned to distinguish nursing from medicine. Without a clear sense of the differences among professions, physicians generally perceive that all health care professionals are available to assist them in implementing their medical care plans. Such physicians have difficulty breaking through their stereotypes.

If and when physicians and other health care colleagues understand the essence of nursing, they will be more likely to support effective nursing care by directly asking for, listening to, and carrying through with nurses' recommendations. This collegial relationship is especially important when nurses work with sick persons in hospitals. Dramatic things happen when physicians, nurses, and other professionals understand one another's roles and work collaboratively. Conditions are created wherein persons with health needs use their own strengths and resources as full participants and responsible agents in their own healing. Tasks related to the medical care plan provide a means and context wherein nurses use their judgments to help people take the best possible care of themselves as whole persons.

Technical procedures become powerful tools in building the trust and conveying the genuine caring that is fundamental to achieving these broader growth and development goals. Such growth will facilitate persons' adherence to medical recommendations, help them develop new attitudes, and reorder lifestyles so as to avoid recurrent illness episodes and maladaptive chronic illness behaviors.

The story of the woman who was admitted to the coronary care unit with a heart attack provides an example.

> Refusing to follow any of the recommended coronary precautions, the middle-aged woman swore so loudly and continuously that doctors and nurses on the evening shift stopped going into her room. They warned the incoming midnight nurses about the "tiger" in room 8.
>
> When the midnight nurse entered the client's room to take her blood pressure, the client renewed her verbal tirade. The nurse deliberately conveyed her acceptance by listening without interrupting, maintaining a soft facial expression throughout. Suddenly, the client stopped swearing. Reaching for the nurse's arm, she commented on her kindness in not leaving the room. When the nurse assured her that she was "worth being kind to," the distraught woman began to cry. Out poured the heartache and grief associated with her husband's sudden death one month before. "What was the point of following doctor's 'orders' when there was no reason left to go on living?" Her nurse continued listening, occasionally sharing a perspective on loss and grief from her theoretical base.
>
> Only minutes later, the client had identified for the nurse what would help her continue her grieving without harming herself physically. She wanted her Bible and a radio to listen to her husband's favorite music; she asked to see her daughter whom she had rejected for bringing her to the hospital against her will.
>
> Early that morning the physician read the nurse's recommendations and the brief theoretical rationale that she included in her charting. He gladly bent the rules of the special unit, commenting on how helpful the nurse's perspective was in helping him to avoid taking the client's anger personally and in renewing his confidence to work again with this woman. He voiced appreciation for the team approach. Three days later, a fast-recovering woman—free of complications and already transferred to the less intensive unit—told her former midnight nurse, "I learned so much that night. About myself, about grieving. . . ."
>
> She also stated that her relationship with the physician was providing opportunity for growth. This growth was not dem-

onstrated by the fact that, as someone said, "The tiger turned into a pussycat." Rather, as she herself put it, "The doctor and I are good friends now. He stops by just to visit and we are sharing many ideas. I'm learning from him and he says he's learning from me, too!"

It is not the physician's responsibility to understand nursing intuitively or to grant nurses spontaneous professional status and respect. Our responsibility in practicing nursing to its full potential is clear. Physicians cannot be expected to change their perspectives on nursing until nurses, themselves, learn to label, describe, and document nursing care that is demonstrably different yet significantly complementary to medicine.

The Consumers

Consumers, like physicians, have difficulty articulating the essence of nursing when they perceive that their nurses are not clear in their own minds. Consumers have always sought nurses because they have wanted personalized, holistic health care. Nurses, however, have devalued the unique care they provide, have often provided it without compensation, have rarely labeled it, and have often sought medical approval of it. As a result, the consumer, too, learns to discount or ignore its value.

It is our experience that when we value, label, and describe nursing, the consumer validates it enthusiastically. Consumers seek our assistance, are willing to pay for it, and recommend us to others. When we ask them what we do that is helpful, they typically say: "You seem to understand." "You care about me, not my illness." "You are there when I feel down." "You are so good with my family and that really helps me a lot." These comments have come from clients in varied settings, both in the hospital and in the community. Let us give you an example.

A client was hospitalized with an acute medical problem. She was extremely ill, required a temporary double-barreled colostomy, had repeated infections requiring several incisions and drainage operations, and remained in the hospital for three and one-half months. She had the usual multiple tubes (intravenous

infusions, nasogastric suctioning, catheters, drains) and extensive pain. After discharge, she arrived at the nurse's door one
evening with a gift to express how much she appreciated the
care she had received. When she commented that this nurse had
been her favorite and had made it possible for her to get better,
visions of "the nurse efficient" flashed through the nurse's
mind; she knew this woman was trying to say that the nurse had
been wonderfully gentle when she irrigated her wounds and
packed in the fine-mesh gauze; that injections had been pain-
less; that the nurse had always been on time for IV fluids, ensur-
ing that she wouldn't have to be "poked" again. Eager to confirm these perceptions, the nurse asked this woman how she
had been helpful. Imagine the surprise when the woman did
not mention one of these nursing functions! Indeed, she said,
"You seemed to care. You would come in and be with me, and
sometimes when I didn't have the energy to talk you seemed to
know that. You held my hand when they drew my blood. You
gave me lots of encouragement by pointing out what I could
do, rather than always talking about what was wrong. You just
seemed to care."

This consumer shares experiences with many others who can
also describe the nurse's special role in helping them to get better.
Take, for instance, the woman who was "comatose" in the intensive
care unit who returned much later to tell students that she would
not be alive today had she not sensed such remarkable empathy and
caring on the part of the nurses. Our clients have helped us understand and articulate our beliefs about nursing—its uniqueness and
its contributions to the health care of individuals and society at large.
In our many years of nursing, we have never had a client say that we
were valued because we gave good medical care, but many have commented on our nursing capabilities!

Unfortunately, there are other consumers who have had experiences with nurses who didn't have the time and energy to provide
nursing care but instead spent their time assisting the doctor to carry
out his medical plan. These consumers may have been treated gently
and with empathy, but still they are unable to state that they received
care that was explicitly directed at anything but the condition or the
disease. Some consumers are not even this lucky. They have had
nurses who were mean and bored and who couldn't wait to go home.
These individuals tend to reinforce the stereotypes of nurses and

nursing that exist today. Again, the problem lies in our inability to be clear, precise, and absolute about our profession.

As we change our approach to communicating who and what we are, we can expect our consumers to become more open and specific about what they receive and most value from their professional nurses. When this happens, our media image will change. Rather than being projected as the sweet, kind pixie who helps Dr. X or as the stern, heavy-set, controlling, gruff nurse who throws visitors out of the patients' rooms, we will be projected with an image that will delight most nurses. In fact, it might be the image that drew many of us into the profession to begin with! When nurses are asked why they wanted to be nurses, many respond with some variation of the comment, "I like people and I wanted to help them." Before we can expect to see this image of nursing projected by the public, our consumers, we must develop a rationale for why holistic nursing is important to the care of the individual and give ourselves permission to practice it.

The Nurses

Nurses themselves contribute to reinforcing old stereotypes. This happens when good nurses practice their nursing intuitively, sometimes even furtively (1)*, and do not proceed to identify systematically and describe explicitly what it is they do that health care consumers value so much. Because of its heavy nurturing component, such nursing is "taken for granted" or equated with common sense. As a result, nurses do not justly credit either themselves or their chosen profession with the enormous benefits they generate. This idea bears repeating. Nurses very often deliver what is distinctly nursing care; simultaneously, they devalue their nursing because they often discount their most powerful interventions. This is partly because they cannot fit such "common sense" within a deliberate, comprehensive framework for the delivery of nursing care (2).

Because they are missing the deep satisfaction that comes from theoretically based nursing, some nurses settle for the meager reward of being commended as helpers and handmaidens to physicians (3). Some pursue an ultimately hollow approval of their competence in handling the complicated equipment used today. Still others content themselves with the limited satisfaction of receiving praise for the

*Numbers in parentheses refer to notes at the end of the chapter.

advanced knowledge of medicine they have acquired since their days as students. They neglect the holistic, self–care, and health aspects of nursing and flounder instead in a single etiology, cause-and-effect approach to problem solving focused on the diagnosis and treatment of injuries, diseases, and disorders (4).

While a cause-and-effect, problem–solving approach may be appropriate for the practice of medicine, nurses using this approach tend to ignore or pay only lip service to the omnipresent psychosocial factors in disease causality, treatment, and health promotion. Such nurses often lack the professional self-image and self-esteem that come from being validated by consumers and nursing colleagues rather than their medical colleagues. Lacking a coherent nursing paradigm, they have difficulty providing client–centered, purposive nursing care. They are rarely able to explain the essence of their practice in a clear, concise, consistent, and comprehensive way. If they disagree with their medical colleagues about approaches that will best serve the patient's interest, they lack a persuasive rationale to elicit respect and action-oriented support for their nursing recommendations. Frequently, these nurses become bored and disillusioned with nursing. Many of them leave the profession; others continue to "work" but feel drained by the end of the shift. They are rarely heard detailing the "joy of nursing."

CONCEPTIONS OF THE NURSE–DOCTOR–CONSUMER TRIAD

Relationships among the nurse, doctor, and consumer have changed over time. We believe that these relationships can be represented as shown in Figure 1-1. Figure 1-1(a) depicts the nurse who perceives herself as a "helper" to the physician. This nurse operationalizes nursing within the framework of the physician's orders. Although these "orders" are really the doctor's medical care plan, this nurse nevertheless perceives them as orders for her to follow as she provides patient care. Such a nurse does not identify or articulate a legitimate, autonomous relationship with the health care consumer. Perhaps nursing was practiced by the majority within this model at one time.

Figure 1-1(b) depicts the situation in which the nurse provides autonomous but not collaborative care. This nurse recognizes and declares a legitimate relationship with her client, while acknowledging the physician's relationship with the patient. Figure 1-1(c) de-

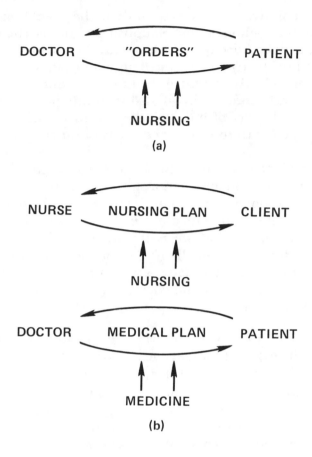

(a)

(b)

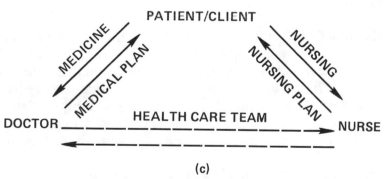

(c)

FIGURE 1-1   The nurse–doctor–consumer triad

picts collaborative care as described in the preceding pages. The nurse enjoys an autonomous relationship with her client and a professional, collaborative relationship with the physician.

Currently many nurses vacillate among these models because they have not clearly identified the essence of nursing and they have not labeled, described, or articulated its components. When we enter an era in the history of nursing wherein nurses label, describe, and articulate the focus, function, and goals of nursing, we will be true professionals.

You will note that the representations in Figure 1-1 have specified a physician–patient relationship and a nurse–client relationship. This was done intentionally, since we believe that a nurse will not have a relationship with a *patient* if and when she practices professional nursing. Instead, she will work with a *client*. Clearly, some physicians also work with clients but most tend to have patients instead. We anticipate that many of you are asking, "What's the difference between a patient and client?" We have chosen to define the two concepts as follows:

A *patient* is one who is given aid, instruction, and treatment with the expectation that such services are appropriate and that the recipient will accept them and comply with the plan.

A *client* is one who is considered to be a legitimate member of the decision-making team, who always has some control over the planned regimen, and who is incorporated into the planning and implementation of his or her own care as much as possible.

Examples of the difference might be helpful. Consider the individual who experienced some chest pain radiating to his left shoulder. He visited his physician and was assessed and diagnosed as having angina. The doctor informed him that he didn't really have any major organic problem, but that he must lose weight, quit smoking, and reduce his stress level to prevent one. This patient was not included in these prescriptions; instead, he was told what steps he must follow.

Subsequently, the same individual called for nursing care. He stated that he knew he had too much stress, but that was part of his life. It was embedded in his job and his home life, and he couldn't give those up. He had tried to quit smoking, and on those occasions had found himself eating more. Furthermore, the very thought of not smoking made him tense, and when he dieted, he smoked more. Here, then, we have a *patient* who was trying to quit smoking, lose weight, and decrease his stress—in short, altering his entire lifestyle to an extent he found overwhelming. When this individual was treated as a *client*, it became clear that he could only manage some of these "orders" at a time and that he had to make the decision whether or not he could manage any of them. The next step was to explore the nature of his stressors so that he might reorganize (not give up) his activities so that they caused less stress and then to discover how he might proceed. He finally decided that he could reorganize his lifestyle (somewhat) and that he could go on "just a little diet." He stated that he was not ready to give up smoking, but maybe he would later, if he lost some weight first. He said that he would feel better about himself if he lost weight, that he would look better and feel better physically. Therefore, this was his first priority.

Within a few weeks he had lost enough weight that he decided to cut back on his cigarettes as well. He continues now to decrease his smoking habit, has lost weight, and does not experience any chest pain. He says that he feels better, is more active than ever, and one day will soon "dump" the cigarettes altogether (5).

Clients are distinguished from *patients* by their active participation in plans for their improved health. As nurses build on an assumption that the client ultimately knows and controls what will help him or her, they will not automatically reject a client who does not "comply with" a recommended medical regime. *Patients are told* that they should take certain medications for their hypertension (for example); *clients are asked* what they think caused their hypertension and what they think will help remedy the problem. Clients are provided with information about various ways to handle these perceived causative factors if they can't readily think of possible solutions of their own. Even so, they have the right to make informed decisions—including the decision that none of the options is appropriate—and the right to choose to do nothing or to suggest another option. Clients are not automatically rejected for making such decisions. Patients, on the other hand, are at great risk of rejection for making them.

Working with *patients* implies that the health care provider is expected to know what's best; working with *clients* implies an understanding that the consumer knows what's best, what will help him or her gain an optimal state of health. Our goal is for nurses to work with clients. Physicians may also choose to do this; that is not our concern as nurses. In our experience, it seems that most physicians are socialized to interact with patients rather than with clients. Although this has also been true for nurses, we contend that holistic health care can only be practiced through an interactive, interpersonal process with a client (6). We appreciate that many nurses who treat their consumers as clients refer to them as patients. This is not a problem for us, as long as those nurses can clearly specify nursing. The important factor is what the nurse is thinking about when she identifies her consumer as a patient or client.

BENEFITS FROM EXPLAINING NURSING

The future of nursing as a viable, self-correcting, and self-governing profession depends on whether nurses, with some help from enlightened clients, will correct the stereotypes and misunderstandings we have discussed in this chapter. Health team members who understand the distinctions among their professions compete less with one another by conscious and unconscious one-upsmanship. Fragmented care that costs clients time, energy, money and unnecessary suffering will decrease. This will prevent many of the crises that, despite our best intentions, we create for clients. Freed from contending with superimposed crises, clients will have more energy to heal faster, cope adaptively, and learn how to take care of themselves according to their true capabilities. Nurses' time and energy will be released to help clients build upon—not merely survive or endure—their immediate experiences.

As nurses raise colleagues' and clients' awareness of their specific contributions, we can openly and directly draw on one another's expertise in a spirit of genuine interdependence. We will *value* our differences in educational preparation and experience because they help us meet goals that no single discipline can reach alone. The client will be included in our processes, adaptively using the control he or she has always ultimately held, even when we fancied otherwise.

When we know who we are and what we do well, and can *say* it boldly and clearly, we will practice our profession with pride and confidence. We will describe, compare, contrast, correlate, predict, and prescribe the elements of nursing in a naturally evolving personal participation in significant nursing research.

Finally, as a natural outcome of all this, nurses, who comprise the largest single body of health care professionals in our society [numbering over 1,600,000 (7)] will affect the political process in both private and public sectors to preserve and promote the kind of nursing valued by receivers and care givers alike.

SUMMARY

Distinct differences among the health professions exist. Nurses, especially, have not differentiated and articulated their unique expertise to themselves, their fellow professionals, and their clients. Nurses often provide quality care intuitively and simultaneously discount it when they have no comprehensive theory and paradigm within which to structure their specialized nursing knowledge and practice.

The development of the profession is also affected by unfavorable stereotypes and by power relations in health care situations based in a view of nursing as subservient to and dependent on medicine. Consumers are frequently treated as *patients* who are passive, rather than as *clients* who participate actively in plans for their own care when deliberately nurtured to that end.

Nursing will thrive as a unique and valued profession when nurses present a theory and rationalistic model for their practice, correct misleading stereotypes, locate control with clients, and actively participate in processes for political change.

NOTES

1. A nurse friend recalls holding a dying patient in her arms after closing the door to hide her actions. And who among us has never "slipped in" a special visitor, pet, favorite food, or an extra swallow?

2. Thomas Huxley once said, "Science is nothing but organized common sense"; and G. K. Chesterton remarked, "Nothing is so elusive as common sense."

3. This is an unfortunate state since theoretically based nursing can be documented and validated easily by measuring intervention effectiveness. Discovering a degree of effectiveness provides the nurse with the positive reinforcement needed to enjoy nursing.

4. This single etiology, cause-and-effect approach to problem solving that focuses on the diagnosis and treatment of diseases, injuries and disorders is often referred to as the "medical model." While nurses also use a problem-solving approach, our focus is not the diagnosis and treatment of disease and disorder but on helping persons holistically.

5. As we go to press, this client has stopped smoking, feels better than he has in years, and is as active as ever.

6. We include the adjective "interactive" because we wish to stress the active participation of both nurse and client in this interpersonal process or relationship between them.

7. Secretary of Health, Education and Welfare, *Second Report to the Congress, March 15, 1979 (revised), Nurse Training Act of 1975*, DHEW Publication no. (HRA) 79-45, Hyattsville, Md.: Division of Nursing, Health Resources Administration 1979, Table 5, p. 114.

Toward a Philosophy of Nursing

OVERVIEW

Although we have inherited barriers that impact on our ability to practice professionally, we have also inherited assets or driving forces, including definitions of nursing. In this chapter we review some published definitions of nursing, noting themes that past and present nursing leaders have held in common. We also briefly consider exciting developments in contemporary nursing.

We encourage you to reflect on nursing's solid heritage in the light of these newer developments. We offer two illustrations that may assist you in considering further developing and refining your own philosophy of nursing.

HISTORICAL FORMULATIONS: COMMON CONCEPTS OF NURSING AGGREGATED

Many classic definitions may be taken from the large body of existing literature. Leaders since the time of Florence Nightingale have attempted to describe the unique aspects of nursing and to relate them to the needs of their contemporary culture. The following pages contain quotations from several of these perceptive and courageous promoters of professional nursing.

As you skim over and think about the various definitions of nursing on the following pages, you will note that over the decades of nursing's formal history as a profession certain common concepts have recurred with slight differences in wording and priorities. The key words have been boldfaced in an effort to assist you in spotting these recurrent themes.

[Nursing puts] us in the best possible conditions for Nature to restore or to preserve health—to prevent or to cure disease or injury. . . . **Health** is not only to be well but to be able to **use well every power we have** to use. Sickness or disease is Nature's way of getting rid of the effects of conditions which have interfered with health. It is Nature's attempt to cure—we have to help her. Partly, perhaps mainly, upon nursing must depend whether Nature succeeds or fails in her attempt to cure by sickness. Nursing is therefore to **help** the **patient** to **live.** Training is to teach the nurse to help the patient to live. Nursing is an art, and an art requiring an organized practical and scientific training. (1)

Florence Nightingale, 1893

Nursing is rooted in the needs of humanity and is founded on the ideal of **service**. Its object is not only to cure the sick and heal the wounded but to bring **health** and ease, rest and comfort to **mind and body,** to shelter, **nourish,** and protect and to minister to all those who are helpless or handicapped, young, aged, or immature. Its object is to prevent disease and to preserve health. Nursing is, therefore, linked with every other social agency which strives for the prevention of disease and the preservation of health. The nurse finds herself not only concerned with the care of the **individual** but with the health of a **people.** (2)

Bertha Harmer, 1922

Nursing requires the application of scientific knowledge and nursing skills and affords the opportunities for constructive work in the care and relief of patients and their families. . . . Modern nursing is by no means limited to the giving of expert physical care to the sick, important as this is. It is more far reaching, including as it does, **helping** the **patient** to adjust to unalterable situations, such as personal, family and economic conditions, teaching him and others in the home and in the community to **care for themselves,** guiding him in the prevention of illness through **hygienic living,** and helping him to use the available community resources to these ends. (3)

Hester Frederick and Ethel Northam, 1938

Nursing is a significant, therapeutic, **interpersonal process.** It functions co-operatively with other human processes that make **health** possible for **individuals** in communities. In specific situations in which a professional health team offers health services, nurses participate in the organizations of conditions that **facilitate** natural ongoing tendencies in human organisms. Nursing is an educative instrument, a maturing force, that aims to promote forward movement of personality in the direction of creative, constructive, productive, personal, and community **living.** (4)

Hildegard Peplau, 1952

Nursing is primarily **assisting** the **individual** (sick or well) in the performance of those **activities contributing to health,** or its recovery (or to a peaceful death) that he would perform unaided if he had the necessary strength, will, or knowledge. It is likewise the unique contribution of nursing to **help** the individual **to be independent** of such assistance as soon as possible. (5)

Virginia Henderson, 1955

Nursing is perhaps best described as the giving of direct **assistance** to a **person,** as required, because of the person's specific inabilities in self-care resulting from a situation of personal **health.** Care as required may be continuous or periodic. **Self-care** means the care which all persons require each day. It is the personal care which adults give to themselves, including attention to ordinary health requirements, and the following of the medical directive of their physicians. (6)

Dorothea Orem, 1959

Nursing is a service to **individuals** and to **families;** therefore, to society. It is based upon an art and science which mold the attitudes, intellectual competencies, and technical skills of the individual nurse into the desire and ability to **help** people, sick or well, **cope** with their **health** needs, and may be carried out under general or specific medical direction. (13)

Faye Abdellah, Irene Beland,
Almeda Martin, Ruth Matheney, 1960

Any individual nurses another when he carries, in whole or in part, the burden of responsibility for what the **person** cannot yet or can no longer do alone. [Nursing] offers **whatever help** the patient may require for **his needs to be met,** i.e., for his **physical and mental comfort** to be assured as far as possible while he is undergoing some form of medical treatment or supervision. (7)

Ida Jean Orlando, 1961

Nursing aims to **assist people** in achieving their **maximum health** potential. Maintenance and promotion of health, prevention of disease, nursing diagnosis, intervention, and rehabilitation encompass the scope of nursing's goals. (8)

Martha Rogers, 1961

. . . to **facilitate** the **efforts of the individual** to overcome the obstacles which currently interfere with **his ability** to **respond** capably to demands made of him by his condition, environment, situation, and time. (9)

Ernestine Weidenbach, 1964

Nursing is an **interpersonal process** whereby the professional nurse practitioner **assists** an **individual** or family to prevent or **cope** with the **experience** of illness and suffering and, if necessary, assists the individual or family to find meaning in these experiences. (10)

Joyce Travelbee, 1966

The nurse participates actively in every patient's environment and much of what she does **supports** his **adaptations** as he struggles in the predicament of illness. Nursing intervention means that the nurse interposes her skill and knowledge into the course of events that affects the patient. Thus, nursing intervention must be founded not only on scientific knowledge but specifically on recognition of the **individual's** organismic **response** which indicates the nature of the adaptation taking place. . . . When nursing intervention influences the adaptation favorably, or toward renewed social **well-being,** then the nurse is acting in a therapeutic sense. When the nursing intervention cannot alter the course of the adaptation—when her best efforts can only maintain the status quo or fail to halt a downard course—then the nurse is acting in a supportive sense. (11)

Myra E. LeVine, 1969

Nursing is a **process** of action, reaction, interaction, and transaction, whereby nurses **assist individuals** of any age and socioeconomic group to meet their basic needs in performing **activities** of **daily living** and to **cope** with **health** and illness at some particular point in the life cycle. (12)

Imogene King, 1971

Nursing is a means to **help** people whose actual or potential deviations from health have inpaired their ability to **cope** with some aspects of **daily living.** Nursing care may be aimed at preventing the initial or further deviations from health, at restoring or enhancing the ability to cope with daily activity, and at maintaining or sustaining the **person's capacities** through a **health** problem. These services may be provided independently of other health professions or in collaboration with them. (14)

Pamela H. Mitchell, 1973

All nursing activity will be aimed at **promoting man's adaptation** in his physiological needs, his self concept, his role function and his interdependence relations during health and illness. (15)

Sister Callista Roy, 1976

[Nursing] is **assisting persons** with their **self-care practices** in relation to their state of **health.** (16)

M. Lucille Kinlein, 1977

The nurse leaders quoted above have defined nursing not only to direct our attention toward both the means and the end goal of the process of nursing but also to identify the focus of nursing. If we take the concepts we emphasized for you and list them together, we note that the list results in a rather complete definition of nursing. Collectively, they say nursing is to

>assist persons
>>with their responses to health and illness states
>>with their self-care practices in relation to their health
>>(with their coping and adapting)
>>to achieve a state of (optimum) wellness
>by way of an interpersonal process.

With such an encompassing view of nursing over the years laid before us, we might complete the picture by raising the important questions, "What's different now?" or "What's new in the modern profession of nursing?" Let's briefly turn to some thoughts along these lines.

MODERN NURSING: NURSING CONCEPTS AND SCIENTIFIC RESEARCH

As with any developing profession in society, we have grown in our understanding of some of the scientific theories underlying skills and judgments that we have developed (often intuitively) over the years. While the major concepts of nursing have existed across time providing a foundation for nursing practice, they now form bases for nursing research.

Through research we are learning more about how our ability to relieve or diminish fear and anxiety affects the musculature of the arterioles of the body to lower (or raise) blood pressure, the musculature of the bronchioles to ease breathing, and the balances of hormones that raise resistance to infection and promote rapid healing. (17)

We are beginning to study scientifically the suggestion that when nurses promote a sense of positive expectation in clients we free our clients to produce their own internal biological tranquilizers and influence critical regulatory hormones and immune system responses via a chain of events initiating in the hypothalamus (18). This augments the body's continuous drive toward health—the internal biochemical and electrical interchanges that result in homeostasis, or what some have called homeodynamism.

As health scientists continue to develop research methodologies suitable to multifactored, naturalistic research settings, we are acquiring statistical support for heretofore strictly intuitive practices: classic nursing interventions as simple as handholding (19), a mellow tone of voice (20), a measured pause (21), a touch, a hug (22), or permission to cry (23). Research has provided evidence to support the notion that one's perception that he or she is being helped is often as powerful a remedy as an externally prescribed agent (24). Our experience suggests that these interventions are frequently essential for successful health-directed goal attainment.

When nurses give people the benefit of this kind of purposive nursing, interacting with people to meet their interrelated needs as complete thinking, feeling, and behaving persons, they may or may not be simultaneously performing manual skills or procedures. We will have more to say about the use of technical procedures in nursing in Chapters 8 and 11 and Part IV.

The answer to our question "What's new in nursing?" (or "What's different about modern nursing as compared to the nursing described by nurse leaders across time?") is simply that we are working more aggressively toward validating the simple, intuitive humanistic interventions valued by our predecessors. This body of knowledge that describes and explains our practice provides a base for increasingly effective professional judgments. It allows us to predict outcomes and write prescriptions for the care of our consumers.

MERGING THE OLD WITH THE NEW: TOWARD YOUR OWN PHILOSOPHY

We believe it is important for you to synthesize the concepts common to all nurses that have developed in various ways at various times in history. From your synthesis you can further derive your own philosophy of nursing, a philosophy you can comfortably describe in your own words, both to yourself and to others. Such conceptualizations will serve as a valuable guideline in your study and practice of nursing. You may at different times choose slightly different ways to express your philosophy of nursing, depending on whom you are addressing and the related circumstances. (We do this, as we show in Chapter 3.) The important point is to help yourself, the public, and your fellow professionals to keep nursing goals in view. These are the goals implicitly or explicitly held in common by all nurses, regardless of differences in approach or methodology, regardless of the age, sex, condition, or location of their clients. The issue, then, is to keep constantly in mind how nursing differs from other professions.

Table 2-1 might help you in achieving this goal. We considered how human beings living in society have developed professions in response to their perceived needs and noted how they have simply, yet effectively, given names to these professions that clarify their different, special contributions. You may agree that we can feel justly proud of our name and its derivation from the word "nurturing."

TABLE 2-1   Some Professions That Have Emerged in Response to a Social Need

Sometimes simply looking at a word enables us to draw on the unconscious collective wisdom of social beings who develop professions in response to human needs.

Profession	Social Need
lawyer	*law* and legal advising
pastor	spiritual *shepherding*
physician	*physical* mending
nurse	*nurturing*
teacher	*teaching*

Two situations may be helpful in illustrating some of the points we have made in this chapter and in Chapter 1. The first illustration shows the usefulness of using a conceptual paradigm in the context of a simple, common hospital nursing situation. The second recalls an experience one of us had which exemplifies a dynamic process of stating one's philosophy of nursing.

Illustration 1:   A Paradigm in Action

At 2:00 A.M. a hospitalized person tells a midnight nurse emphatically that his most pressing need is for a period of unbroken rest, free of any interruptions, including the early morning blood pressure reading routinely prescribed by the physician, as well as the physician's visit on early morning rounds. After a thoughtful exchange of data and health information with his nurse, the patient requests that the nurse intercept all possible disturbances during the next six hours. In full support, based on her holistic analysis of factors (not merely the biophysical), the nurse agrees to carry out his request. She omits the A.M. blood pressure reading and posts a notice at the door to the patient's room to check with her before knocking or entering. She herself makes noiseless periodic checks throughout the night to assure herself of his well-being.

When the physician arrives in the morning and wants to

wake the client, he hears a clear description from the nurse of the data and principles underlying her nursing judgment. Depending on opportunity and need, the nurse might choose to help the physician understand further the complementarity of her nursing judgments and interventions with his own medical care plan. Quite reasonably, the physician in this situation will learn some nursing from the nurse, just as nurses learn medicine while working with physicians. Each, however, practices his or her own profession. As a result of the nurse's interventions, the client awakens spontaneously, refreshed and much improved, exulting in his "first real rest" since his admission. His adaptation energy is now available for healing and restoration.

Illustration 2:   An Explanation in Process

We were sitting at the breakfast table one bright, sunny morning with old friends we had not seen for several years. "Just what kind of nursing do you do?" asked Dave, referring to my venture into private nursing practice.

I noted that he did not immediately equate a "private practice" of nursing with private duty nursing, as another friend had done earlier the same month. Dave knew I nursed people who were not necessarily sick or confined to room or bed. Nor had he asked "What do you do?"—a question often posed by those who are baffled by the idea that there exists a need for nursing outside a medical or hospital setting.

I smiled inwardly in renewed awareness of how often I am asked such questions. I began explaining for the fourth time in as many weeks, "Well, let me put it this way." I noticed I was gearing up to use slightly different wording again.

"I help people, Dave, in any way that they perceive I can, to meet a need or want that will enable them to take better care of themselves. I pay attention not only to any physical care needs, but to simultaneous mental, emotional, and spiritual ones, too. Humans are whole persons, Dave, and what happens at one level affects the other parts of us as well."

I saw the familiar nodding of heads, bobbing immediate agreement, as Dave and his wife listened attentively. This spurred me on: "Because of my broad-based nursing education, it's my special expertise and privilege to meet the whole person's needs in an integrated way. I start with whatever concerns that person most.''

Since they were still with me, I gathered steam. "Whole persons need access to a care giver who 'holistically' nurtures—or *nurses*—their self-care. I look right away for strengths that are there, and do everything I can to nurture even the smallest ones, like fanning a small spark to see the joy of a warm, brightening flame burst forth.''

Dave chimed in enthusiastically. "Yes, that's what Loretta and I appreciated when you came to our house that day. You saved Mark's life, you know. We always felt that. You knew what to do when you helped bring his temperature down. But most of all, you cared. About Loretta and me, too, and the terrible distress we were in. We'll never forget!''

The episode Dave referred to had occurred 28 years before. What Dave and Loretta seemed to have realized then (as I hardly did myself during those tender beginning practice days) was just how that caring for them, the concerned parents, interlaced with and facilitated the positive physical response their infant son gave to my care of him. As our conversation continued, Dave supported what he called this "new concept" of nursing. I replied that I thought the means and places of delivering nursing care might be different, but the essence of that care had always been the unique expertise and concern of nurses and nursing.

This episode exemplifies how each nurse who possesses a nursing philosophy can contribute to educating and reinforcing a public who (in our experience, at least) is happy to have put into words what they have known but haven't been able to express for themselves. The public has an influential voice in our legislative halls and regulatory departments where society's decisions are being made. This last example particularly demonstrates why a nurse should have several consistent versions of her philosophy of care. If we are to communicate effectively, we must learn to communicate within the context of each respondent's interest and understanding.

It goes almost without saying that a nursing philosophy must be congruent with a personal philosophy of life if it is to be useful. Without such congruence, a nurse would not be comfortable operationalizing the philosophy of nursing. For, clearly, nursing is an interpersonal process that cannot be specified without considering the characteristics of the nurse herself as well as the focus of the care she offers.

SUMMARY

We have highlighted common themes from nursing's respectable heritage. Our past emphasis on nursing as a practice discipline joins a current concern to develop the science of nursing. The latter is evolving from an increasing amount of nursing research as well as research from other disciplines. Studies describing mind–body relationships have particular relevance to holistic nursing practice and support heretofore intuitive practices.

We have encouraged you to develop a personal philosophy of nursing consonant with concepts identified by nurse leaders and with yourselves. As we learn to express our nursing philosophy and what we do with clients in personal, concise definitions and theoretical formulations, these precise articulations will help our colleagues, our clients, and the public to understand nursing goals and the distinctness of nursing from other health professions.

NOTES

1. Florence Nightingale in *Selected Writings of Florence Nightingale*, compiled by L. Seymer (New York: Macmillan, 1954), pp. 334–35.

2. Bertha Harmer, *Textbook of the Principles and Practice of Nursing* (New York: Macmillan, 1922), p. 3.

3. Hester Frederick and Ethel Northam, *A Textbook of Nursing Practice*, 2nd ed. (New York: Macmillan, 1938), p. 3.

4. Hildegard Peplau, *Interpersonal Relations in Nursing: A Conceptual Frame of Reference for Psychodynamic Nursing* (New York: Putnam's, 1952), p. 16.

5. Bertha Harmer, *Textbook of the Principles and Practice of Nursing*, 5th ed., rev. by V. Henderson (New York: Macmillan, 1955), p. 4.

6. Dorothea Orem, *Guides for Developing Curricula for the Education of Practical Nurses* (Washington, D.C.: Government Printing Office, 1959), pp. 5–6.

7. Ida Jean Orlando, *The Dynamic Nurse–Patient Relationship* (New York: Putnam's, 1961), p. 5.

8. Martha Rogers, *Educational Revolution in Nursing* (New York: Macmillan, 1961), p. 23.

9. Ernestine Weidenbach, *Clinical Nursing: A Helping Art* (New York: Springer, 1964), pp. 14–15.

10. Joyce Travelbee, *Interpersonal Aspects of Nursing*, (Philadelphia: F. A. Davis, 1966), pp. 5–6.

11. Myra E. LeVine, *Introduction to Clinical Nursing* (Philadelphia: F. A. Davis, 1969), p. 10.

12. Imogene King, *Toward a Theory for Nursing: General Concepts of Human Behavior* (New York: John Wiley, 1971), p. 22.

13. Faye Abdellah, Irene Beland, Almeda Martin, and Ruth Matheney, *Patient-centered Approaches to Nursing* (New York: Macmillan, 1960), p. 24.

14. Pamela H. Mitchell, *Concepts Basic to Nursing* 2nd ed. (New York: McGraw-Hill, 1973), p. ix.

15. Sister Callista Roy, *Introduction to Nursing: An Adaptation Model* (Englewood Cliffs, N.J.: Prentice-Hall, 1976), p. 18.

16. M. Lucille Kinlein, *Independent Nursing Practice with Clients* (Philadelphia: Lippincott, 1977), p. 23.

17. Hans Selye, *The Stress of Life*, 2nd ed. (New York: McGraw-Hill, 1976).

18. H. Laborit, "On the Mechanism of Activation of the Hypo-thalmo-pituitary-adrenal Reaction to Changes in the Environment (The Alarm Reaction)," *Resuscitation* 5 (1976): 19-30. Kenneth Pelletier, *Mind as Healer, Mind as Slayer* (New York: Dell Pub. Co., Inc., 1977), p. 53.

19. James Lynch, "The Simple Act of Touching," *Nursing* 78 (June 1978), 32-36.

20. M. Smart and R. Smart, *Infants, Development and Relationship*, 2nd ed. (New York: Macmillan, 1978), pp. 75-76.

21. Kinlein, M. L., *Independent Nursing Practice with Clients* (Philadelphia: Lippincott, 1977), p. 66.

22. P. MacMillan, "Spacing and Touching and Hugging," *Nursing Times* (1981), 788-90. P. Heidt, "Effect of Therapeutic Touch on Anxiety Level of Hospitalized Patients," *Nursing Research* 30 (1981): 32-37.

23. W. Frey, II, and others, "Effect of Stimulus on the Chemical Composition of Human Tears," *American Journal of Opthalmology* 92 (1981): 559-67.

24. A dramatic instance of repeated tumor exacerbation and re-gression in relation to a client's faith in his treatment is told in Charles Garfield, ed., *Stress and Survival, The Emotional Realities of Life-Threatening Illness* (St. Louis: C.V. Mosby, 1979), pp. 5-6.

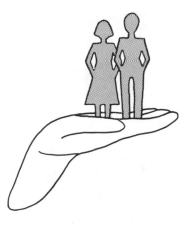

II

A THEORY-BASED PARADIGM FOR NURSING

In Part I we considered factors that influenced our ability to practice professional nursing. We encouraged you to consider some of these factors and then develop a philosophy of nursing that can be used to guide your practice.

In this section we present our philosophy and definition of nursing, our theory base, and our paradigm for the practice of nursing. Our philosophy and definition of nursing is in Chapter 3, our theory base is in Chapters 4 through 6, and our paradigm is in Chapter 7.

A Philosophy and Definition of Nursing

OVERVIEW

We developed our philosophy and definition of nursing after several years of in-depth consideration and practice. We owe a great debt to the many theorists who provided us with important insights. Some theorists we studied were not integrated into our model because their ideas were incongruent with our philosophy, theory, and paradigm. You will note that we have not deviated from our professional inheritance, but instead have expounded on concepts laid down through the years, starting with Florence Nightingale.

We have not included our beliefs about the role of medicine because this book is about nursing. Nevertheless, we think that it would be helpful for you to address this issue as you develop your own philosophy. Without a clear notion of how the doctor's role differs from the nurse's role, nurses often have difficulty conceptualizing a philosophy of nursing autonomous from medicine (1).

OUR PHILOSOPHY

We believe that nursing is a process between the nurse and client and requires an interpersonal and interactive nurse–client relationship that is independent of the doctor–patient relationship. It does not necessarily include or exclude a collaboration between nurse and doctor. That is, nursing occurs both *independent* of a doctor–patient relationship and *in collaboration with* a doctor who has an established doctor–patient relationship with the nurse's client.

Our philosophy of nursing encompasses several major concepts that include both the role of the nurse and human nature. These concepts are depicted in Figure 3-1 and are described below. Concepts that relate to human nature pertain to *all* humans; thus they apply to nurses, doctors, and clients. These concepts do not relate to the role of the doctor as a *professional*. As stated above, we have not addressed this phenomenon in this book (2).

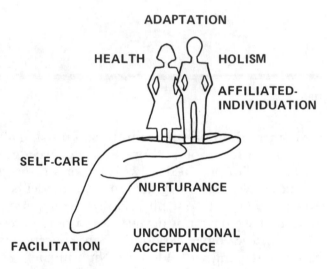

FIGURE 3-1   Concepts in our philosophy

CONCEPTS RELATING TO HUMAN NATURE

Holism

Human beings are holistic persons who have multiple interacting subsystems (see Figure 3-2). Permeating all subsystems are the inherent bases. These include genetic makeup and spiritual drive. Body, mind, emotion, and spirit are a total unit and they act together. They affect and control one another interactively. The interaction of the multiple subsystems and the inherent bases creates holism. *Holism* implies that the whole is greater than the sum of the parts.

Figure 3-3 symbolically depicts the "whole person." *Wholism* is defined as the state in which the whole is equal to the sum of the parts. Wholism suggests that man is an aggregate of the biophysical, psychological, social, and cognitive subsystems with inherent bases throughout; it does not imply dynamic relationships among these subsystems. Since we have stated that we believe that humans are holistic (not merely wholistic), Figure 3-2 best represents our beliefs. From this perspective, conscious and unconscious processes are of equal importance. Most useful changes result from a blend of both.

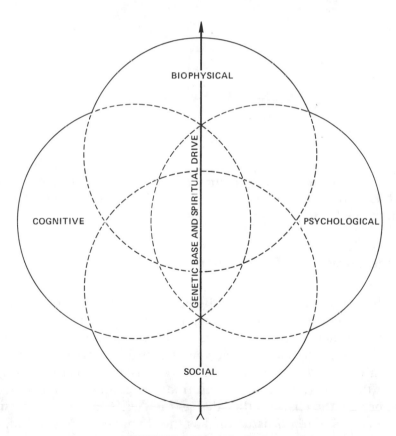

FIGURE 3-2   A holistic model

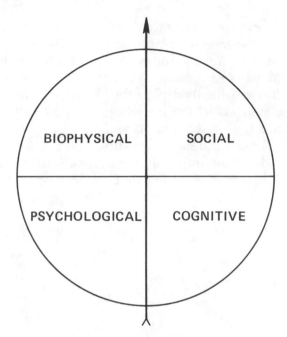

FIGURE 3-3   A wholistic model

Health

Health is a state of physical, mental, and social well-being, not merely the absence of disease or infirmity (3). It connotes a state of dynamic equilibrium among the various subsystems.

Lifetime Growth and Development

Individuals are born with an inherent desire to fulfill their self-potential. Our needs are species wide and are related to both survival and growth; they motivate our actions. Each human is also born with a capacity for growth and development over the entire life span. People are always and invariably in a continuous movement or changing state. If they are given accurate information, emotional support, and assistance for the changes they desire, they will make good decisions for themselves. *Growth* is defined as the changes in body, mind, and spirit that occur over time. People can become larger and stronger; their bodies, ideas, social relations, and so forth differ at different points in time. Growth implies ongoing integration of these various facets of a person. Growth facilitates development. *Development* is the holistic synthesis of the growth-produced increasing differentiations in a person's body, ideas, social relations, and so forth. Growth and development promote health.

Affiliated-Individuation

Individuals have an instinctual need for *affiliated-individuation*. They need to be able to be dependent on support systems while simultaneously maintaining independence from these support systems. They need to feel a deep sense of both the "I" and the "we" states of being and to perceive freedom and acceptance in both states (4).

Adaptation

There is an innate drive toward holistic health, growth, and development. Self-healing, recovery, renewal, and adaptation are all instinctual, despite the aging process or inherent malformations. Stressors in life exist at all times. They exert their positive and negative effects on the person according to the meaning that the individual attaches to them and according to the resources the person has to adapt to them. Illness and stressful experiences of all kinds have the potential to eventually and ultimately provide overall growth and life enhancement. One person's threat is another's challenge or opportunity. Individuals need stressors; health and happiness depend on learning to cope constructively by mobilizing resources to contend with stressors.

Adaptation occurs as the individual responds to external and internal stressors in a health and growth–directed manner. Adaptation involves mobilizing internal and external coping resources. No subsystem is left in jeopardy when adaptation occurs.

Maladaptation occurs when an individual copes with a stressor within one subsystem by taxing energies from another. For example, if a person confronts a social stressor but is unable to engage constructive coping methods or mobilize appropriate resources to contend with the stress caused by the stressor, the person might tax his or her biophysical subsystem for coping resources. This would result in biophysical subsystem vulnerability since the subsystem would be at a higher risk if additional stressors were to emerge. There would be a diminished supply of resources available to call forth for the purpose of coping with such stressors. Biophysical health problems such as hypertension might develop. Thus, one subsystem is in jeopardy due to unresolved stressors in another; this is maladaptation.

Self-Care: Knowledge, Resources, and Action

At some level a person knows what has made him or her sick, lessened his or her effectiveness, or interfered with his or her growth. The person also knows what will make him or her well, optimize his or her effectiveness or fulfillment (given circumstances), or promote his or her growth. We call this *self-care knowledge*. *Self-care resources* are two-fold, internal and external. *Self-care action* is the development and utilization of self-care knowledge and self-care resources. Through self-care action the individual mobilizes internal resources and acquires additional resources that will help the individual gain, maintain, and promote an optimal level of holistic health.

CONCEPTS RELATING TO THE ROLE OF NURSE

Facilitation (5)

The nurse is a *facilitator*, not an effector. Our nurse–client relationship is an interactive, interpersonal process that aids the individual to identify, mobilize, and develop *his or her own strengths*.

Nurturance

Nursing care can only be delivered through interpersonal interactions in the context of an ongoing relationship. Nurturance fuses and integrates cognitive, physiological, and affective processes, with the aim of assisting a client to move toward holistic health. Nurturance implies that the nurse seeks to know and understand the client's *personal model of his or her world* and to appreciate its value and significance for that client from the client's perspective. Having thus *modeled* the client's world, in subsequent interactions the nurse thoughtfully and purposefully *role-models* that world with the client so that the client can grow *healthier* (6).

Unconditional Acceptance

Being accepted as a unique, worthwhile, important individual—with no strings attached—is imperative if the individual is to be facilitated in developing his or her own potential. The nurse's use of empathy helps the individual learn that the nurse accepts and respects him or her as is. The acceptance will facilitate the mobilization of resources needed as this individual strives for adaptive *equilibrium*.

A DEFINITION OF NURSING

Now that we have defined the concepts incorporated in our philosophy of nursing, it is fairly simple to develop a definition of nursing. We are not so presumptuous as to propose that this definition is unique or markedly insightful. It does, however, provide us with a clear understanding of our professional practice. Here again you will note the integration of concepts previously described by nurse leaders over the years. Specifically, this definition is our attempt to articulate what nursing is, how nursing is accomplished, and the goal of nursing from our perspectives.

This definition of nursing does not specify the "tasks" of nursing, since we believe that tasks are merely the means to an end (7). In brief, then:

> *Nursing* is the holistic helping of persons with their self-care activities in relation to their health. This is an interactive, interpersonal process that nurtures strengths to enable development, release, and channeling of resources for coping with one's circumstances and environment. The goal is to achieve a state of perceived optimum health and contentment.

Several abbreviated versions extracted from the above definition have been helpful in our own dialog with others about our individual practices. Each version is consistent with our more comprehensive definition but shorter.

Nursing is the nurturance of holistic self-care.

Nursing is assisting persons holistically to use their adaptive strengths to attain and maintain optimum bio-psycho-socio-spiritual functioning.

Nursing is helping with self-care to gain optimum health.

Nursing is an integrated and integrative helping of persons to take better care of themselves.

SUMMARY

We have briefly defined the concepts embedded in our philosophy of nursing and have given a definition of nursing based on these concepts. We have addressed our assumptions about human nature, the role of the nurse, and the nature of nursing. In essence, we have said that the human is a holistic, health-oriented being who strives for growth and development when facilitated in the continuous process of adaptation. The individual is the primary source of information concerning his or her needs and resources. The individual's inherent needs, including a need for affiliated-individuation, motivate the individual's behavior. Nursing is an interactive, interpersonal process that facilitates persons in attaining growth, development, and holistic faith. Growth and development are best advanced by nurturance and empathetic unconditional acceptance.

The remaining chapters in Part II will present the theoretical bases from which we have derived our theoretical formulations. The final chapter presents our paradigm for the practice of nursing.

1. Below are some thoughts on how clinical medicine and clinical nursing differ. You will easily add to these distinguishing features.

Clinical Medicine	Clinical Nursing
Focuses on biophysical subsystem: diagnosing and *treating disease* and curing the person.	Focuses on holistic (multisystem) *person:* assessing unmet needs—taking all subsystems into account—and the capacity of the individual to mobilize resources for coping, thus *caring* for the *person* in the person's self-care efforts.
Stresses problem identification and problem solving.	Stresses strength identification and builds from that point.
Harmonizes biophysical needs and biophysical treatment demands.	Harmonizes the whole person's self-care activities.
Cannot begin *treatment* until a diagnosis is made.	Nursing *care* begins at first moment of contact when nursing expertise may be needed to ease the client's expression of what brings him or her for care and what the client already knows will help him or her to achieve an optimum state of health. (At some level, those who are sick know what has made them ill and what can help them get well.)
Can often be given without requiring an interpersonal relationship.	Can only be given through an interactive, interpersonal process.
Prescriptive functions are specific to the problem presented, for example, a wound or infection.	Prescriptive functions are specific to the *prime expressed concern* of the client. They fall into broader categories or *aims* that are designed to facilitate self-care by activating, restoring, or augmenting coping resources. Effective *caring* by the nurse then generalizes out through efforts of the client to beneficially affect other aspects of the person's total well-being.
Seeks to decrease trouble and weakness.	Seeks to increase comfort and strengths.

Clinical Medicine	Clinical Nursing
Tends to focus on *current* state of being with an emphasis on physiological measures of wellness.	Considers the normal developmental sequence with a focus on *growth* and highest level function. Seeks to promote growth and development of the multisystem person.

2. Below are excerpts from the Occupational Regulation Sections of the Michigan Public Health Code. You will note that there are significant differences in our purposes. While other states' practice acts may differ from these, you will probably find that there is a different focus in the goals of the two professions.

Part 170. Medicine: section 17001 (c)
"Practice of medicine" means the diagnosis, treatment, prevention, cure, or relieving of a human disease, ailment, defect, complaint, or other physical or mental condition, by attendance, advice, device, diagnostic test, or other means, or offering, undertaking, attempting to do, or holding oneself out as able to do, any of these acts.

Part 172. Nursing: section 17201 (a)
"Practice of nursing" means the systematic application of substantial specialized knowledge and skill, derived from the biological, physical and behavioral sciences, to the care, treatment, counsel, and health teaching of individuals who are experiencing changes in the normal health processes or who require assistance in the maintenance of health and the prevention or management of illness, injury, or disability.

3. World Health Organization, "Constitution of the World Health Organization," *The Chronicle* (1947): 29-43.

4. Sister Teresa Marie McIntier, "Theory of Interdependence," in Sister Callista Roy, ed., *Introduction to Nursing: An Adaptation Model* (Englewood Cliffs, N.J.: Prentice-Hall, 1976), pp. 291-302.

This concept may at first sight seem to be identical to Sister Teresa Marie McIntier's concept of interdependence. McIntier discusses the theory of interdependence which she defines as, "The comfortable balance between dependence and independence in relationships with others" (p. 291). Our concept of affiliated-individuation shares with the concept of interdependence the notion of the individual's need for affiliation (dependence). But the two concepts differ in their meaning of independence. Independence for McIntier contains the idea of the need for an individual to "accomplish tasks on his own without others" (p. 293). In our opinion, this meaning of independence includes the satisfactory working through of several of Erikson's developmental stages. Independent *task achievement* suggests that the individual has acquired a sense of autonomy, initiative, and industry. Our notion of individuation is different; we see individuation as akin to acquiring a sense of autonomy, as in Erikson's stages. The individual is separate from a significant other with a will of his own and control over himself (independence) while concurrently sensing trust that he can and will be taken care of (dependence).

5. The order of these three concepts (facilitation, nurturance, and unconditional acceptance) does not suggest that we perceive one is more important than another. We believe that each is of equal importance in establishing a trusting, functional relationship.

6. The concepts of *modeling* and *role-modeling* are explained fully in Chapter 7.

7. What we mean by this is that technical skills are extremely important "tools" that can be used to establish a trusting, functional relationship with your client. We believe that the important factor is why you do what you do. If you give medications, insert catheters, suction, start intravenous fluid, take blood pressures, and so forth, *because the doctor orders them*, then you are focusing on the doctor's orders and working toward medical goals, not your own professional goals.

4

Theoretical Bases: How People Are Alike

OVERVIEW

The question "How does one describe and explain how people are alike?" has directed our thinking for several years. Nurses generally talk about the uniqueness of their clients, but we must also consider how people are alike if we are to develop theory bases for the practice of nursing. Here we present our thoughts about how people are alike and review theory bases related to these concepts. You will note that we continue to follow our philosophical beliefs presented in Chapter 3.

HOLISM

As we sought answers to our question "How are people alike?" one fact seemed to stand out. Humans are essentially alike in their biophysical makeup. Nurses study anatomy, physiology, biochemistry, and microbiology and are then able to describe how most people are "made up" biophysically. Most people have an immune response system, a stress response pattern (endocrine system feedback loop), respiratory system, cardiovascular system, renal system, and so forth. All of these can be described with a common language (1). Nurses need to know what is normal and how people compare in the biophysical subsystem; they need to be able to label and describe how these phenomena are alike in all humans. Without this knowledge, nurses are unable to detect deviations from normal which may signal the need for sickness care. Without this information nurses are unable to know when their clients are healthy.

People are not only alike in their biophysical subsystem responses, but they are also alike in that they are holistic. A person is not just a head and a body, a thinking mind without feelings or physiological needs. The notion that the human is a biophysical, psychosocial, and spiritual being was introduced earlier in this volume. This concept encompasses the belief that the human is a holistic, multisystem being. Also postulated was the idea that a relationship exists between mind and body. When needs are not met within one subsystem (to some significant extent, and from the person's perspective), a potential exists for the individual to draw energy from another subsystem in order to maintain himself or herself (maladaptation). As a result, individuals have a propensity to become physically sick when experiencing psychosocial stressors or emotionally distressed when experiencing biophysical stressors. Every practicing nurse has many examples of this mind-body relationship.

Consider the individual who experiences multiple psychological stressors who begins to sleep poorly and eat unwisely and soon comes down with a common cold or bladder infection. Or consider the ulcer patient who starts to bleed after having a disagreement with a significant other, the person who has dyspnea and pulmonary edema on the heels of "bad news," the patient who is disappointed because no one visits and then seems to regress in recovery, and the person who gets a simple headache when things "pile up."

Research also supports the relationship between mind and body. A survey conducted among students in Puerto Rico revealed a tremendous surge in the use of health clinic facilities during examination periods (2). A study of nursing students conducted in Ann Arbor, Michigan, showed that a significant relationship exists between feelings indicating distress and the use of health care facilities (3). Others have also shown these relationships between mind and body (4).

More subtle examples supporting the linkage of subsystems come from patients themselves who tell nurses the things that helped them most in recovering: "You were there when I needed you." "You held my hand during that painful treatment." "It was your smile that carried me through." "Your voice was so soothing." "You said it was OK to ask questions." "After you explained it, I understood." And so on.

We humans often express feelings through our bodies when for some reason we do not feel safe or we do not know how to state or describe our feelings directly. It is not without reason that our popular language abounds with such phrases as "cold feet," "scared stiff," "heavy hearted," "hot headed," "tickled pink," "sick with disgust," "can't swallow that," "it's a pain in the neck," "I've got a lump in my throat," "she makes me sick," "he gives me a headache," "scared silly," "drives me crazy," and so forth. Feelings seem to affect our physiology and our physiological state seems to affect the mind. Clearly, most of us can say that there are times when we have experienced a physiological problem resulting in psychological distress, and vice versa. Humans are alike in that they have a mind–body relationship.

LIFETIME GROWTH: BASIC NEEDS

As we continued to search the literature for help with the question "How are people alike?" we were struck with the correspondence of Abraham Maslow's (5) formulation of the growth principle and theory of human needs to our own clinical observations. Maslow states that all people want to be the best that they can possibly be; unmet basic needs interfere with holistic growth whereas satisfied needs promote growth. We had also observed that all humans seem to have basic needs which, if not attended to, can very often lead to the initiation or aggravation of physical or mental distress and illness. These needs are both physiological and psychological in nature, and in many cases they precede the need to learn. Finally, these needs seem to drive (motivate) our behaviors.

Examples of the innateness of these needs can be drawn from the practice of almost every nurse. If you have asked the average heart attack patient, "What has been the problem and what do you think caused your illness?" you have probably heard such typical responses as: "Too much pressure at work" or "Things are not going well at home." Embedded in these responses are statements about unmet psychosocial needs that have resulted in unmet physiological needs, for surely a heart attack is an unmet physiological need.

Maslow has described these needs as existing in a hierarchy. Needs on the lower level of the hierarchy must be satisfied to some degree before the higher level needs emerge. These needs and their hierarchical relationship with one another are shown in Figure 4-1.

A building has been used to illustrate the hierarchy, because we believe that the similarity between Maslow's theory and our beliefs can be symbolized by the building of a strong structure. If the foundations (basic needs) are strong (needs are well satisfied), the base will stand strong and be able to resist the distress of the environment over time, just as the human will grow to be strong and cope adaptively when his or her needs are met over time.

Imperative in this concept is the notion that *basic needs are only met when the individual perceives that they are met.* A mother (or other care giver) may try very hard to satisfy these needs but, no matter what, until the individual perceives that they are satisfied, they are not. For example, the infant lacking the normal bacilli in the intestine may have some difficulty digesting milk. Although the infant may gain weight, he or she may also have colic. The infant will have great dif-

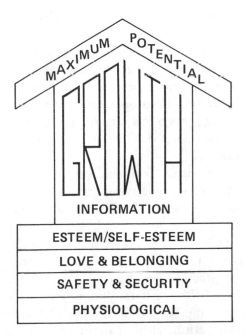

FIGURE 4-1   Maslow's hierarchy of needs

ficulty in perceiving that his or her physiological needs are satisfied when his or her body "hurts." Such a state of affairs can even result in the infant's perception that safety and security needs have not been satisfied, since infants learn to feel safe and cared for through the satisfaction of physical needs. Following through to the greatest extent, this same infant could perceive that his or her love needs are also not met, since it is the care giver who meets all needs at this stage in life. Finally, if the problem were prolonged, it is conceivable that a negative cycle between mother and infant would be initiated. Mother tries hard for a long time; nothing seems to help; mother quits trying so hard; the problem gets worse. Clearly, the situation could have long-standing implications.

We have taken the time to expand on this example because of its implications for the nursing process. Nurses often find themselves ignoring difficult, demanding patients who seem impossible to satisfy. Once the nurses have tried everything, they simply do not know what else can be done. As with the mother–infant relationship, the same can happen in the nurse–client relationship: the more the patient is ignored, the worse the situation gets. If, however, we can keep in mind that *all human beings have basic needs that can be satisfied, but only from within the framework of the individual,* we might direct our care more purposefully and remember to incorporate the consumer as a client instead of as a patient.

If we take Maslow's ideas about survival and growth needs seriously, we can understand why when any basic survival needs are unmet there is little point expecting a person to progress beyond his or her preoccupation with those deficits or to deal with the growth needs that invest life with meaning. Even less can this person be expected to "find his or her place in the universe," or reach his or her fullest potential for health and happiness.

This simple relationship between survival and growth needs has huge implications for nurses who try to teach a person something while that person's energies are being depleted by an unsatisfied basic need (or needs), not only the first level biophysical needs but also the constant, concurrent needs for safety, affection, and respect. Although we nurses generally pay lip service to these ideas, we often forget to apply them deliberately in practice.

In our zeal for professionalism, patient education has become an important part of nursing. Within the context of Maslow's theory, however, providing information without first assessing whether or not the basic needs have been met may be very distressing for the individual.

Many people will have difficulty comprehending, let alone mastering, what is being taught. In fact, there is evidence (6) to suggest that *didactic teaching* itself, when arbitrarily done, *can become an added stressor* that increases feelings of helplessness and hopelessness. These feelings may be out of proportion to the reality of the situation, but, nevertheless, they are real feelings and can cause real physiological responses!

The fundamental issue related to education of clients is whether there is a need to know or a fear of knowing. Simply stated, Maslow believed that a person has a need to know for two reasons. First, there is the need to gain information for "its own sake, for the sheer delight and primitive satisfaction of knowledge and understanding per se. It makes the person bigger, wiser, richer, stronger, more involved, more mature" (7). This kind of knowledge meets growth needs and helps the individual develop self-potential.

Second, there is the "need to know," described by Maslow as the search for information or knowledge as a method of coping with fear and anxiety. In this case, the acquisition of knowledge meets safety and security needs. This need to know is associated with survival instead of growth. Maslow also talked about the fear of knowing. Individuals sometimes avoid knowledge in order to feel safe and avoid anxiety. These individuals have unmet safety and security needs and perceive additional information as a further threat to their safety.

When we educate prematurely (without assessment of true readiness and the effect of current stressors), people may continue to signal their crucial unmet basic needs by acting out related feelings, usually those of helplessness, inadequacy, or hopelessness, but often those of fear, frustration, and fury. Such acting out may take the form of withdrawal, apathy, unexpected dependency, or clinging; conversely, it may take the form of contrary, aggressive, antisocial behavior. In our practices, we have often worked with persons who were "not ready" even to talk about their disease or illness and its demands on them until they were fully convinced we cared about helping them with what *they perceived* were more basic concerns.

This principle also applies to children who have a natural eagerness to learn once their basic needs have been satisfied. Thus, a child who is having learning difficulties needs the benefit of a teacher who understands basic-need theory. Consider one such child whose plight is brought to a nurse's attention. A nurse using this theory would immediately assess for evidence of unmet basic needs and engage or recommend that the teacher engage interventions designed to meet those needs while simultaneously offering the suggestible child a verbalized, constructive, positive expectation for the future. Assume a youngster whose home life is relatively stable. During a time of physiological and psychological good feeling (as when coming in from recess), this child might be asked a quick question about a pre-recess lesson, for example, a multiplication problem. If the child answers incorrectly, the teacher gives the correct answer along with a cheery hug and the simultaneous suggestion: "Won't it be neat when you'll be able to tell me the correct answers?" This prevents reinforcing the child's potential for internal decision making in the category of "I musn't make a mistake" (learning instead to "play it safe") or "I must avoid displeasing teacher by what I do or say" (in order to retain respect). Rather, the child is freed to reach some personalized form of the conclusion: "I'm liked (loved) for *me*, not because I'm right (or smart, or perfect). Teacher's right! I do like learning."

Whatever stressors might contribute to the child's problem, the relationship with the teacher will certainly not be the cause of incomplete involvement in the teaching–learning enterprise, withdrawal, or aggressive behaviors. When esteem and self-esteem are protected and promoted, the way will be paved for the child to "go on to the joy of learning." The traditional nursing emphasis on existing strengths is implicit in this example. The strengths are the *responsiveness* of the child, plus a projection of the nurse's own conviction that a physically well child who is feeling secure, accepted, and esteemed will indeed learn cognitive material appropriate to the child's age level if reasonable flexibility in the timing for achievement is maintained. One way to build "the use of an existing strength" into a situation wherein a child does not even offer a response would be for the teacher to give the answer with a warm smile and hug and then ask the child to restate the answer. The suggestion for future positive performance may then take such a form as, "Now you *know*, Jack! You've got it, you're learning. Learning is fun!"

The principle is to create an atmosphere of total, unconditional acceptance through some genuine praise or acknowledgment of accomplishment (in this case, for imitation, because that was the strength of the moment). Because this acceptance results in lowered anxiety (i.e., satisfies needs for belonging and esteem), the child's capacity to absorb, retain, self-motivate, or self-direct is invited to emerge. The sequence of events may also be viewed as a form of indirect suggestion wherein the smile and squeeze, with tonal emphasis, become anchors for recapturing the moment's profoundly good feeling (arising from the building blocks of the child's multisensory perception of the moment) for repeated associations of the good feeling with the child's developing learning capabilities (8). Finally, projecting the individual into the future with the *positive* expectation that the child can and will learn when the child is ready satisfies needs for security, belonging, and esteem.

Implicit in this entire discussion of basic needs is the notion that anxiety is secondary to unmet needs. We believe that this is the case, but there is often a difference between anxiety related to basic-need deficit and anxiety related to growth needs. Generally, basic-need deficit results in a threat to the individual, while lack of growth-need satisfaction generally provides a challenge for the person. Both cause anxiety, but threatening anxiety utilizes more resources than does challenging anxiety. Although we are not certain, we think that challenging anxiety prepares one for growth activities, and that threatening anxiety promotes a defensive activity state (9).

LIFETIME DEVELOPMENT: PSYCHOLOGICAL STAGES

Erik Erikson offered another perspective in answer to the question "How are people alike?" (10). This time our observations of clients and our own growing families coincided with those of a published theorist. Erikson describes eight stages of psychosocial development through which we all progress. Each stage represents a developmental task or decisive encounter resulting in a turning point, a moment of decision between alternative basic attitudes (for example, trust versus mistrust or autonomy versus shame and doubt). As a maturing individual negotiates or resolves each age-specific crisis or task, the individual gains enduring strengths and attitudes that contribute to the character and health of the individual's personality in his or her culture. Erikson calls these attitudes *virtues*. We have listed the tasks and associated virtues and strengths in Figure 4-2. Again, as with Maslow's hierarchy, these tasks are listed from the bottom up rather than from the top down. This is to illustrate the need to start at the base and work up, rather than to work from the top down, for solid structures start with solid foundations.

Erikson says that each of these critical characteristics of psychosocial development is systematically related to all the others. While varying in tempo and intensity of resolution, they all "depend on the proper development in the proper sequence" of each, and each "exists in some form before its critical time normally arrives." Moreover, "they

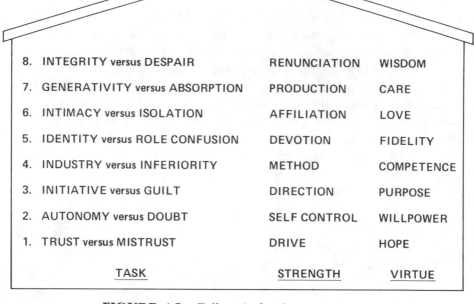

TASK	STRENGTH	VIRTUE
8. INTEGRITY versus DESPAIR	RENUNCIATION	WISDOM
7. GENERATIVITY versus ABSORPTION	PRODUCTION	CARE
6. INTIMACY versus ISOLATION	AFFILIATION	LOVE
5. IDENTITY versus ROLE CONFUSION	DEVOTION	FIDELITY
4. INDUSTRY versus INFERIORITY	METHOD	COMPETENCE
3. INITIATIVE versus GUILT	DIRECTION	PURPOSE
2. AUTONOMY versus DOUBT	SELF CONTROL	WILLPOWER
1. TRUST versus MISTRUST	DRIVE	HOPE

FIGURE 4-2   Erikson's developmental stages

must all exist from the beginning in some form, for every act calls for an integration of them all" (11). People who normally negotiate the critical step or turning point of each and all preceding stages in sequence have at their disposal strengths and resources essential for effective, age-appropriate functioning that includes observable behavior, introspective experiencing, and unconscious inner states. According to Erikson, young adults are theoretically working toward resolution of the crisis or task of intimacy versus isolation. Yet it is very possible to find 50-year-olds who are still "working through" or completing that chronologically more youthful stage of psychosocial development. Indeed, a 50-year-old may need to complete or resolve a task of a much earlier stage in life (such as one involving the task of trust versus mistrust or autonomy versus shame and doubt). Although we use the expression "completing an earlier developmental task" to describe the acquisition of fundamental psychosocial functional skills by a person, we agree with Erikson that this does not imply that a "once and for all" or lasting solution obviates all new inner conflicts and automatically mediates changing life conditions in this flawed and unpredictable real world. The utility of Erikson's theory is the freedom we may take to view aspects of people's problems as "uncompleted tasks." This perspective provides a hopeful expectation for the individual's future since it connotes something still in progress. Compare this to the perspective that one is "fixed" in a state of development, *is* schizophrenic, obsessive-compulsive, passive-aggressive, a denier, manipulator, and so forth. This kind of labeling promotes a sense of permanence, a sense that, no matter what, this person will never be anything but passive-aggressive.

Many of you will recall nurses who have referred to patients as "the gallbladder in 246B" or "the grouch in 15A." These nurses often treat people as gallbladders, or as grouches, not as humans who have basic, unmet needs. Labeling individuals in this manner tends to fragment care; it interferes with the goal of facilitating holistic persons in acquiring the help they want and need from us.

LIFETIME DEVELOPMENT: COGNITIVE STAGES

Another way to think about how people are alike is to consider their cognitive development, that is, to consider how thinking develops rather than what happens in psychosocial or affective development. Piaget provided us with insight into this commonality (12). His theory base has four major concepts: schemata, assimilation, accommodation, and equilibration. *Schemata* are the cognitive structures by which individuals adapt to and organize their environment intellectually. You can think of schemata as categories or units of information, that is, as a set. Piaget argues that these structures exist, even though there are no absolute data to support this statement. *Assimilation* is a cognitive process by which the person integrates new perceptual stimuli into existing schemata or patterns. In other words, as the individual acquires more information, the individual integrates that information into existing schemata. *Accommodation* is the establishment of a new schema or the modification of an old schema (or schemata) in order to accommodate new information. *Equilibration* is the balance between assimilation and accommodation. When disequilibration occurs, the individual is motivated to assimilate or accommodate further.

Piaget believed that cognitive learning develops in a sequential manner and he has identified several periods in this process. Essentially, there are four periods: sensorimotor, preoperational, concrete operations, and formal operations. (See Table 4-1.) But within these periods there are several substages.

The sensorimotor period starts at birth and lasts approximately two years. It can be broken down into six substages. The first substage occurs from the time of birth until about one month. During the entire sensorimotor period, the infant is dominated by the physical manipulation of objects and events. During substage one [birth to one month (also known as the *reflexive stage*)], there is no differentiation between assimilation and accommodation. According to Piaget, this substage involves purely reflexive adaptation. Substage two occupies approximately months one to four and is known as *primary circular reactions*. There is a slight differentiation now between assimilation and accommodation. There is repetition of schemata and self-imitation, especially vocal and visual, and reflex activities become modified with experience and coordinated with each other. Substage three occurs from four to eight months and is described as *secondary circular reactions*. Differentiation exists between assimilation and accommodation but they are still overlapped. In this substage the infant repeats actions in order to prolong an interesting observation or experience. The infant is beginning to demonstrate attention and bolder activity (for example, the infant who kicks). Substage four occurs between eight months and one year. This is when coordination of secondary schemata occurs. The child is now beginning to show clear differentiation between assimilation and accommodation and begins to apply the old schemata to new situations; problem solving also emerges. This stage is known as the *coordination of secondary schemata stage*. Substage five, occurring between months 12 and 18, is known as *tertiary circular reactions*. It is a time when ritualistic repetitions of chance schema combinations begin. The child accentuates and elaborates on ritual. The child begins to use trial-and-error experiments in order to see the result and find new ways to solve problems. Substage six, beginning at 18 months and running through the remainder of the second year, is a time of invention of new solutions by mental combinations. It is not until this time that the individual is able to do any symbolic representation. It is only at this time that very primitive symbolic representations emerge. A mental symbol is either imitated, created or both. Symbolic schemata are reproduced outside their context, in other words, outside the environment in which they are learned and used. Thus, there begins a transition between practice play and symbolic play proper.

The second major stage in cognitive development, according to Piaget, is known as the *preoperational period*. This period occurs between the ages of two and seven years. During these years, language is the major tool for cognitive processing and functioning symbolically. The first substage is known as the *preconceptual*. It occurs between two and four years. At this time the child uses representational thought to recall the past, to represent the present, and to anticipate the future. The child is able to distinguish between "signifier" or "signified." The child is extremely egocentric and always uses self as a standard for others. The child cannot think about phenomena from another's perspective; the child cannot understand why the other does not see things the same as he or she does. During the preconceptual substage, categorization is based on single characteristics. The second substage of the preoperational stage, known as the *intuitive stage*, occurs between four and seven years. During this time there is increasing body function. While the child is beginning to see things from another's perspective, for the majority of the time subjective judgments still dominate the child's perception. The child is beginning to be able to think in logical classes, is beginning to be able to see simple relationships, and is able to understand number concepts and more exact imitations of reality.

The third stage of cognitive development according to Piaget is known as *concrete operations*. This generally occurs between the ages of seven and eleven years. At this point mental reasoning processes assume logical approaches to solving concrete problems. The child is able to organize objects and events into higher classes or along a continuum of increasing values. In other words, the child is able to classify experience and develops skills of reversibility, classification, seriation, transitivity, and conservation (13).

The final period in cognitive development is *formal operations*. This period generally emerges between ages 11 and 15. In formal operations the child is able to think logically and manipulate abstract concepts; hypothetical deductive thought processes begin to occur. The child is now able to implement a scientific approach to problem solving and can handle all kinds of combinations of facts in a systematic way. Each level incorporates and integrates processes from the previous level. Schemata are continually added and modified throughout life. Quantitative changes continue to occur throughout the life span, but qualitative changes cease to occur after the development of formal operational thought.

During the formal operations period, the individual lives both in the present and the future, or the nonpresent. The individual is not only

TABLE 4.1   Piaget's Stages of Cognitive Development

Period	Age	Characteristics
Sensori-motor	0–2 years	Thought dominated by physical manipulation of objects and events
Substage 1	0–1 month	Pure reflex adaptations
		No differentiation between assimilation and accommodation
Substage 2	1–4 months	Primary circular reactions
		Slight differentiation between assimilation and accommodation
		Repetition of schemata and self-imitation, especially vocal and visual
		Reflex activities become modified with experience and coordinated with each other
Substage 3	4–8 months	Secondary circular reactions
		Differentiation between assimilation and accommodation, still overlap
		Repeat action on things to prolong an interesting spectacle
		Beginning to demonstrate intention or goal-directed activity
Substage 4	8–12 months	Coordination of secondary schemata
		Clear differentiation between assimilation and accommodation
		Application of known schemata to new situation
		Schemata follow each other without apparent aim
		Beginning of means–ends relationships
Substage 5	12–18 months	Tertiary circular reactions
		Ritualistic repetition of chance schema combinations
		Accentuation and elaboration of ritual
		Experimentation to see the result, find new ways to solve problems
Substage 6	18–24 months	Invention of new solutions through mental combinations
		Primitive symbolic representation
		Beginning of pretense by application of schema to inadequate object
		A symbol is mentally evoked and imitated in make-believe
		A symbolic schema is reproduced

TABLE 4.1 Piaget's Stages of Cognitive Development (Cont.)

Period	Age	Characteristics
		outside of context; thus, transition between practice play and symbolic play proper
Preoperational	2–7 years	Functions symbolically using language as major tool
Preconceptual	2–4 years	Uses representational thought to recall past, represent present, anticipate future Able to distinguish between signifier and signified Egocentric, uses self as standard for others Categorizes on basis of single characteristic
Intuitive	4–7 years	Increased symbolic functioning Subjective judgments still dominate perceptions Beginning ability to think in logical classes Able to see simple relationships Able to understand number concepts More exact imitations of reality
Concrete operations	7–11 years	Mental reasoning processes assume logical approaches to solving concrete problems Organizes objects, events into hierarchies of classes (classification) or along a continuum of increasing values (seriation) Reversibility, transitivity, and conservation skills attained
Formal operations	11–15 years	True logical thought and manipulation of abstract concepts emerge Hypothetical deductive thought Can plan and implement scientific approach to problem solving Handles all kinds of combinations in a systematic way

*From J. Piaget, *The Psychology of Intelligence*, Transl. by M. Piercy and D. E. Berlyne (Totowa, N.J.: Littlefield, Adams, 1973), and *Plays, Dreams and Imitation in Childhood*, transl. by C. Gattengo and F. M. Hodgson (New York: Norton, 1951). Also from J. H. Flavell, *The Developmental Psychology of Jean Piaget* (New York: Van Nostrand, 1963). From C. S. Schuster and S. S. Ashburn, *The Process of Human Development: A Holistic Approach* (Boston: Little, Brown, 1980). Used by permission.

concerned with what is but also with what might be. The individual begins to build systems, whereas prior to formal operations the individual did not theorize or build systems. When in the formal operations or formal thought period, the individual uses theoretical thought.

It has recently been discovered that there are individuals who grow to adulthood without having developed the ability to use formal operations (14). We believe, however, that the sequential stages described by Piaget are species-wide and that individuals who do not develop the last stage of cognitive development have encountered impediments in their learning process.

AFFILIATED-INDIVIDUATION

A fourth way that people seem to be alike is that there tends to be an innate need for humans to attach to one another across the life span. The infant "needs" its mother; the mother "needs" the infant; the husband "needs" his wife; the teenager "needs" his friends, and so forth. But an equally important component of these human relationships is the need for each member to be simultaneously independent of the other person. *Affiliated-individuation* occurs when a person perceives himself or herself as simultaneously close to and separate from a significant other. *Affiliated-individuation is an intrapsychic phenomenon and can occur without being reciprocated.* Interdependence is the mutual relationship between two human beings and is a different phenomenon. (See Chapter 3, note 4.)

Our thinking about affiliated-individuation is based on the work of authors who have described object relations theory. While many have studied these concepts, Winnicott, Kline, Mahler, and Bowlby (15) have provided the vast majority of the literature. Theoretically, the infant incorporates the care giver into his or her world as he or she experiences repeated, positive contact with her. Over time, the infant develops an attachment to the mother. This attachment is crucial for the normal health and growth of the child. As time goes by, the child begins to move toward a separation-individuation process wherein the child develops a sense of autonomy from the mother. During this time the child generally transfers some of his or her attachment behavior to an inanimate object (a transitional object). Winnicott states that this is the child's first "not me" attachment (16). (The attachment to the mother is a symbiotic relationship; therefore, the infant perceives the mother as part of itself.) Typical transitional objects include soft, cuddly blankets, diapers, pillows, or teddy bears.

According to these authors, people also attach to other transitional phenomena throughout childhood, for example, the baseball glove, favorite doll, best dress, or an animal. Research supports the notion that object attachment is vital for adaptive coping (17).

These theorists do not use the term affiliated-individuation and they do not explicitly articulate its significance. Nevertheless, we feel that the concept is implied in some of their writings. Mahler, for example, describes the child's need to be symbiotically attached to the mother and later separated from her while constantly being free to return for "refueling" (18). Affiliated-individuation, then, is a need to be dependent on a significant other while simultaneously enjoying autonomy from that individual. This delightful relationship of independence with dependence is a common need for all humans.

The awareness and reality of separateness implies that any important attachment can potentially be severed. Engel has stated that object loss (this severing of attachment) can be real, threatened, or perceived (19). That is, the loss of the object may not be real but it may be perceived as a loss. Nevertheless, the consequences are the same. A two-year-old child whose mother brings home a new baby may suffer object loss. This toddler, because of his or her developmental stage, could well perceive mother's absence as abandonment and her changed behavior upon return home as rejection. The result: perceived loss of mother from whom the child had not completely separated. Another example would be the adolescent male whose father throws away the tattered old shirt to which the boy has become attached. He also experiences real loss.

Engel states that all loss produces a grief response, whether the loss is real, threatened, or perceived. Grief is a process that occurs in five stages: denial and shock, development of awareness with anger, restitution, loss resolution, and idealization. When the loss is unresolved a state of morbid grieving results (20). The individual continues to grieve for the lost object for a long time (although the individual may suppress awareness of the loss). People in morbid grieving fluctuate between angry-hostile feelings and sad-depressed feelings. They tend to spend time in purposeless activity. Finally, then, people are alike in their innate need for *affiliated-individuation* and in their innate response to loss.

SUMMARY

We have indicated that people are alike in that we are all biophysical, psychosocial beings who want to develop our potential, that is, to be the best we can be. We have basic needs that motivate our behavior, including a drive for *affiliated-individuation*. Growing to our potential proceeds through sequential, predictable stages in life in both the cognitive and psychosocial domains. Every human shares these commonalities, but each person is also unique. In Chapter 5 we will address how people differ from one another.

NOTES

1. Each of you probably has a favorite physiology reference book. Ours is *Human Physiology* by A. Vander, J. Sherman, and D. Luciano (New York: McGraw-Hill, 1975).

2. Unpublished observations collected by one of the authors (Helen Erickson) while living in Puerto Rico and working as Director of Health Services at Inter-American University (1961–1964).

3. An unpublished study of 123 students in the School of Nursing, University of Michigan, Ann Arbor, conducted by Mary Ann Swain, Helen Erickson, Evelyn Tomlin, Mary Hunter, and Christine Boodley (1980).

4. Many scholars have shown such relationships. Among the most well known are Richard H. Rahe, Thomas H. Holmes, Minoru Masuda, L. E. Wolff, and H. G. Hinkle. A few references are listed in the bibliography.

5. Abraham Maslow, *Motivation and Personality*, 2nd ed. (New York: Harper & Row, Pub., 1970).

6. A 1976 study by S. B. Steckel and M. A. Swain supported the conclusion that persons who receive education without assistance in coping were ultimately less healthy or "less improved" over initial measures than those who received no formal teaching at all. See "Contracting with Patients to Improve Compliance," *Hospitals* 51 (Dec. 1, 1977): 81–84.

7. Abraham Maslow, *Toward a Psychology of Being*, 2nd ed. (New York: D. Van Nostrand, 1968), p. 63.

8. For those who may be unfamiliar with the term *anchor*, let us explain. All of our experiences in life are made up of a combination of sensory components: auditory, visual, kinesthetic, olfactory and gustatory. When a single component of an experience "takes us back" to an earlier time in our lives, that component serves as an *anchor* for the experience. Most of us can readily recall an instance in which a distinctive odor, such as that of new-mown grass, has brought to our awareness a full sensory experience from the past, such as helping with Saturday yard work or visiting the park. For more information about anchoring, you may enjoy reading the clear description of Milton Erickson's work given by John Grinder, Judith DeLozier and Richard Bandler in *Patterns of the Hypnotic Techniques of Milton H. Erickson, M.D.*, volume 2 (Cupertino, California: Meta Publications, 1977), pp. 59–71.

9. This theoretical stance is an integration of repeated observations, data collected in the study mentioned in note 3, our integration of Maslow's thoughts on basic- and growth-need deficits, and Lazarus' thoughts on threatening versus challenging stressors. See Richard Lazarus, *Psychological Stress and the Coping Process* (New York: McGraw-Hill, 1966). A secondary source is Sharon Roberts, *Behavioral Concepts and Nursing Throughout the Life Span* (Englewood Cliffs, N.J.: Prentice-Hall, 1978).

10. Erik Erikson, *Childhood and Society* (New York: W. W. Norton & Company, Inc., 1963).

11. _____, *Childhood and Society*, p. 271.

12. The original presentation of these ideas can be found in J. Piaget, *The Origins of Intelligence in Children* (New York: International Universities Press, 1952). A fairly complete, but easy to read, version of these ideas can be found in J. L. Phillips, *The Origin of Intellect: Piaget's Theory* (San Francisco: W. H. Freeman & Company, Publishers, 1969).

13. Table 4.1 will help you review the characteristics of this stage. For a more detailed description of these phenomena, we refer you to Phillips as referenced in note 12.

14. Jean Piaget, "Intellectual Evolution from Adolescence to Adulthood," *Human Development* no. 15 (1972):1-12.

15. Several references are listed in the bibliography at the back of this book. Nevertheless, you will find that John Bowlby's three books, *Attachment*, *Separation*, and *Loss*, provide an extensive and sufficient background.

16. D. Winnicott, "Transitional Objects and Transitional Phenomena: A Study of the First Not-me Possession," *International Journal of Psychoanalysis* 34 (1953): 89-97.

17. Resources to consider are: Harry Harlow and Robert Zimmerman, "Affectional Responses in the Infant Monkey," *Science* 130 (1959): pp. 421-32. Rene A. Spitz, "Anaclitic Depression," *Psychoanalytic Study of the Child* 2 (1946): 313-342. John Bowlby, *Attachment* (New York: Basic Books, 1969). John Bowlby, *Separation* (New York: Basic Books, 1973). John Bowlby, *Loss* (New York: Basic Books, 1981).

18. Although this concept of refueling was first described by M. Furer, it is often associated with M. S. Mahler. We like to think of refueling as synonomous with "getting your battery charged." The child returns to a safe, secure figure in order to rest and store up sufficient energy to venture into the world again. We have all seen the two-year-old who runs away from mama only to quickly return, grasp her leg,

and "refuel." We believe that adults also need to have an affiliation with another human that will help them "refuel."

19. George Engel, *Psychological Development in Health and Disease* (Philadelphia: Saunders, 1962), pp. 293-94.

20. Erich Lindemann, "Symptomatology and Management of Acute Grief," *American Journal of Psychiatry* 101 (1944): 141.

Theoretical Bases: How People Are Different

OVERVIEW

In Chapter 4 we described how people are alike. We presented the notion that humans have many commonalities, all of which can be considered when providing nursing care. We also know that people are different—each person is unique in his or her own way. In this chapter we give attention to how people can be systematically addressed in their uniqueness. We will cover three major themes: a person's inherent endowment, a person's ability to adapt, and a person's model of his or her world.

INHERENT ENDOWMENT

While it may go without saying, we feel the need to comment on how people are different based on their inherent endowment. By this we mean that each individual is born with a set of genes that will to some extent predetermine appearance, growth, development, and responses to life events. This genetic base will influence how the individual meets his or her needs, perceives phenomena, and so forth.

Take, for example, the child who just seems to know how to play the piano while others struggle, practice, and never reach the same level of expertise. There are children who seem to have no difficulty focusing on what is causing them to feel anxious and there are others who always seem to be uncertain. And then there is the child with Grandma's red hair or a great-uncle's funny nose, there is the tall family, as compared to the short, stocky family, and so forth.

In addition to their genetic makeup, individuals have inherent characteristics that influence their health status. These include malformations, brain damage, or other pathophysiological states secondary to birth, prenatal disease, sicknesses, or other factors. Clearly, both genetic and inherited characteristics influence growth and development. They might influence how one perceives oneself and one's world. They make individuals different from one another, each unique in his or her own way.

ADAPTATION

Another way that people are different involves the adaptation process. There are two major ways to think about adaptation. The first is to consider the nature of the stimulus and response as it relates to the individual's ability to mobilize resources to contend with the stressor. The second way to think about adaptation is to consider the difference between stress and distress. While the two ways to think about adaptation are closely related, they are two different issues and need to be considered separately. Each is of great importance when considering how people differ.

Adaptation Potential

We will begin this discussion with a simple statement that a stimulus is something that produces an action or changes an action in an organism. Stated another way, if a stimulus is encountered, a response occurs. The stimulus triggers the response.

Stress is a response that has specific identifying characteristics. When stress occurs secondary to a stimulus, that stimulus can be labeled a *stressor* (1). Selye described the stress response from a biophysical perspective while Engel described it from a psychosocial point of view (2). We have attempted to synthesize the two views. As we were considering these relationships, several critical incidents came to mind. Three of them are described below.

As an impressionable, observant, and inquiring nursing student, one author cared for a 25-year-old man, about to be married, who was admitted for a routine circumcision. He received the usual preoperative preparation, including chest X-ray, EKG, etc., and was seen to be "in perfect health." The night before surgery he was heard to say, "I'm scared to death." Although the remark didn't mean anything to her when it was made, it was burned into her memory when, during surgery the next day, he had a cardiac arrest and died on the table.

A 51-year-old schoolteacher, recently retired, underwent a radical neck resection for known cancer. Two weeks after the surgery was performed she learned to suction herself, feed herself by tube, and change her own dressings. She was making active plans to move into a new home with her husband and enroll in a class to learn esophageal speech. The evening before her expected discharge, her surgeon told her that during the operation the tumor in her neck had been totally removed but that other tumors existed which were not resectable. He told her she had a life expectancy of about nine months to a year. After the well-intentioned surgeon left, the woman immediately slumped into her chair. She refused to eat or suction herself and said simply, "I want to go to bed." Feeling that was indeed what she wanted, the nurse left her alone. Three days later the woman died.

A 34-year-old woman with three children had severe headaches that signaled the presence of a glioma. She was taken to surgery where the tumor was judged inoperable. As she lay in a postsurgical coma, her discouraged surgeon informed her husband, "There is nothing more we can do." Stubbornly refusing that message and mindful of Patricia Neal's successful recovery from a severely disabling stroke, the husband responded, "Oh, yes, there is." "You *will* do radiation and you will do chemotherapy." He stationed himself at the unconscious woman's bedside and maintained a steadfast vigil there. He talked to her, stroked her hand, told her what was going on with their children, shared his plans for their family. "I know you can't respond. It probably makes you feel very bad. But you will be better, and you will be part of our family again." One author recalls that the nurses on the unit, herself included, regarded the husband sympathetically. "Poor fellow. He's taking this so hard. He probably needs his denial for a time." On the fifth day the woman began to stir. Slowly but surely, before the astonished eyes of everyone but the husband, she began to recover. Ultimately, she went home, returning at three-month intervals for follow-up care. A full two years later, the nurse saw the woman for a last visit. The patient was doing very well and had just been informed that her most recent brain scan was normal.

"These things happen" is our common response to explain such mysterious and unexpected occurrences in which people get well when apparently they couldn't and others die for no well-known reason. Older and wiser now, we believe those persons had differences in their ability to mobilize their self-care resources.

The Body.   Hans Selye, called the father of stress theory, has pointed out that people have different abilities to respond to life stressors, depending on what resources they have. He called these resources *adaptation energy* (3). In his experiments with animals, he demonstrated conclusively that a stereotyped group of general physiologic changes occurred in response to various specific stressors. He discovered that this response was triphasic, and he called it the *general adaptation syndrome* (G.A.S.). The stages in Selye's biological stress syndrome were named the alarm reaction, the stage of resistance, and the stage of exhaustion. Stages were further broken down to include shock and countershock phenomena in the alarm reaction and exhaustive stages. You may recall the generalized outcome of movement into the exhaustive stage: enlargement and hyperactivity of the adrenal cortex, shrinkage of the thymus and lymph nodes, and gastrointestinal ulcers. The G.A.S. is shown in Figure 5-1. The stages and related physiological responses in each stage of his G.A.S. are given in Table 5-1.

Selye's identification of the triphasic nature of the body's response to stress provided evidence that the body's adaptability to stressors is finite. Selye compared adaptation energy to an inherited fortune from which we can make withdrawals and noted that there is no evidence to suggest that we can make deposits. It is true that we

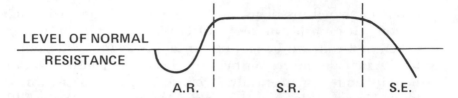

FIGURE 5-1   Selye's General Adaptation Syndrome (G.A.S.). A.R. is the alarm reaction, S.R. is the stage of resistance, and S.E. is the stage of exhaustion. [Hans Selye, *The Stress of Life* (New York: McGraw-Hill, 1976), p. 111. Used with permission.]

have all experienced a resurgence of energy at times, following on the heels of a very draining experience, as if we were borrowing from one or more of several checking accounts we owned to cover a deficit in another. But once the deep reserves of adaptation energy (which Selye compared to long-term investments) have been completely exhausted, the body succumbs to the ultimate effort of constant wear and tear; this is the exhaustive stage. Illness, disease, and even death can result.

Selye was always careful to point out the *positive effects* of stress and stressors too. Consider how we put children into an alarm state purposefully with immunization so that they'll be in a stage of resistance the next time they encounter that same disease-producing organism (stressor). A certain amount of stress can be health promoting, as in this case. But if we give too much of a particular immunizing agent, it will push the child's biophysical subsystem past a stage of resistance to an exhaustive stage which, unless relieved, could ultimately result in death.

The Mind.   People are not, of course, mere physiological organisms. While Selye and other biophysical scientists were working in their laboratories demonstrating the effects of physical stressors such as cold, heat, infection, hemorrhage, and nervous irritation, social scientists, including George Engel, were also observing and documenting stress phenomena in humans. Engel, however, was interested in psychosocial responses to stressors. Building on the work of other keen observers, including Cannon and Schmale (4), Engel placed people into one of two distinct stress categories, depending on their response to a psychosocial stressor (5). These stages were called *fight-flight* and *conservative-withdrawal*. Since then, Seligman (6) and others have described Engel's conservative–withdrawal

TABLE 5-1 Biophysical Phenomena: General Adaptation Syndrome (G.A.S.)

Alarm Reaction		Stage of Resistance	Exhaustive Stage	
Shock	Countershock		Countershock	Shock
depressed nervous system	excretion of epinephrine	normal range systolic pressure	excretion of epinephrine	depressed nervous system
decreased muscle tone	elevated systolic blood pressure	normal range diastolic pressure	elevated systolic blood pressure	decreased muscle tone
hypotension	equal or lower diastolic blood pressure	normal range pulse	equal or lower diastolic blood pressure	hypotension
leucopenia	increased pulse pressure	glyconeogenesis transfer of free fatty acids to triglycerides	increased pulse pressure	leucopenia
eosinopenia	increased pulse rate	protein anabolism	increased pulse rate	eosinopenia
hemoconcentration	glycogenolysis	normal range respiratory rate	glycogenolysis	hemoconcentration
decreased plasma glucose	gluconeogenesis	normal range temperature	gluconeogenesis	decreased plasma glucose
protein catabolism	mobilization of free fatty acids		mobilization of free fatty acids	protein catabolism
hypochloremia	protein catabolism		protein catabolism	hypochloremia
hypothermia	increased respiratory rate		increased respiratory rate	hypothermia
	hyperthermia		hyperthermia	

Based on various textual materials from H. Selye.

state as a helpless-hopeless state. Engel has also described it as a giving-up syndrome.

The Mind–Body Connection.   Considering Selye's general adaptation syndrome and Engel's responses to stressors, we concluded that these phenomena were probably very similar but had been discovered and studied and labeled differently because Selye and Engel had been concerned with a subsystem of the person rather than with the whole person. Conceptually, Selye's alarm reaction seemed to be like Engel's fight-flight response, and Selye's stage of exhaustion was similar to Engel's conservative-withdrawal response.

Since we are concerned with the whole person, we synthesized the two. Our aim was to identify states of coping that would reflect an individual's potential to mobilize self-care resources. We thought that such categorization would help nurses plan interventions more effectively (7). For years nurses have been able to differentiate stress from nonstress states, but have lacked a model that would predict an individual's potential to cope with stress. Thus, our model, the *adaptive potential assessment model* (APAM), which identifies three different coping potential states, provides nurses with new knowledge.

This *adaptive potential assessment model* has three categories which we have labeled *arousal* (A), *equilibrium* (E), and *impoverishment* (I). *Equilibrium* has two possibilities: *adaptive equilibrium* and *maladaptive equilibrium*. Each of the three major states (A, E, and I) represents a different potential to mobilize self-care resources, resources that are biophysical and psychosocial. While *arousal* and *impoverishment* are both stress states, persons in *impoverishment* have diminished, if not depleted, resources available for mobilization. Thus, these individuals are at greater risk when they try to contend with ongoing or new biophysical and psychosocial stressors. People in *equilibrium* have a good potential for mobilizing coping resources. The phenomena of each state are shown in Table 5-2. The APAM differs from Selye's G.A.S. in several ways. First, an individual can move directly from *arousal* to *impoverishment*, depending on the individual's ability to mobilize resources needed to counteract or contend with the stressors encountered. This possibility is shown in Figure 5-2. The second difference is that we show a dynamic relationship among the stages of the APAM rather than a unidirectional process across the stages of the GAS (Figure 5-1). This dynamism is shown in Figure 5-3. Movement among the states is influenced by one's ability to cope (with ongoing stressors) and the presence of

TABLE 5-2 Adaptive Potential Assessment Model:
Phenomena Specific to Each State

Equilibrium (adaptive)
  normal blood pressure reading
  normal pulse
  normal respiration
  expression of marked hope and positive expectations
  absent or low feelings of tenseness and anxiousness
  normal motor-sensory behavior
  absent or low feelings of fatigue, sadness, and depression

Arousal:
  marked feelings of tenseness and anxiousness without feelings of
    fatigue, sadness, and depression
  elevated motor-sensory behavior
  elevated systolic blood pressure
  elevated pulse
  elevated respiration
  high score for verbal anxiety

Impoverishment:
  marked feelings of tenseness and anxiousness with feelings of fatigue,
    sadness, and depression
  elevated verbal anxiety
  elevated motor-sensory behavior
  elevated blood pressure
  elevated pulse
  elevated respiration

new stressors. Since one's ability to mobilize resources is influenced by nursing interventions, movement from *impoverishment* to *equilibrium* is possible within the APAM. Finally, the APAM differs from Selye's G.A.S. because APAM represents a holistic perspective whereas Selye's is a biophysical stress response syndrome.

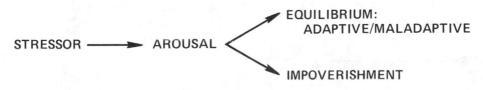

FIGURE 5-2 Adaptive potential assessment model

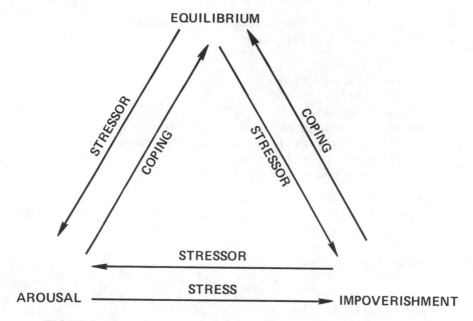

FIGURE 5-3   An illustration of the dynamic relationship among the states of the adaptive potential assessment model

Previous research has supported the hypothesis that individuals could be reliably classified according to the *adaptive potential assessment model* (8). Further study of these states is underway at this time. We continue to explore the potential relevance of phenomena other than those shown in Table 5-2. For instance, we are as interested in the impact of the feelings that represent a state of activeness and happiness on one's sometimes concurrent feelings of fatigue, sadness, and depression. Further, we wonder whether there is an important difference between physical fatigue and emotional fatigue as these bear on coping potential and health status. Our continued research should lead to a better understanding of these relationships. Nevertheless, while we continue our exploration of phenomena that discriminate the states of coping potential, one from the other, we are confident that these states already can be distinguished by considering the phenomena identified in Table 5-2.

Stress Versus Distress

As we continue to consider the phenomena of adaptation, but this time from a slightly different perspective, let us assume that a stimulus produces a response. With this in mind, we must question when the stimulus is a stressor that mounts a stress response that is potentially healthy and growth producing and when it becomes a distressor that drains or depletes the individual of energy, possibly resulting in maladaptation and illness. Again we turn to the literature for insights.

Selye stated that a stressor becomes distressful when it is prolonged or exceeds the individual's ability to mobilize adaptation energy. The result from Selye's perspective is a disease of distress (9). Lazarus has given us another way to consider the problem of stressful versus distressful stimuli. While not using the exact words stressor or distressor, Lazarus has stated that the way an individual responds to an event or occurrence depends on whether the individual perceives it challenging or threatening (10). Within this context, we can assume that a psychological stressor could be conceptualized as an event or occurrence that is perceived as a challenge and that a distressor is an event or occurrence that is perceived as a threat. Physiological stressors might be those wherein the individual has adaptive energy available to contend with the stressor, while distressors diminish or deplete the store of adaptation energy.

In summary, then, a *stressor* is a stimulus that is experienced as challenging or one that mounts an adaptive response; a *distressor* is a stimulus that is experienced as threatening or one that mounts (either directly or indirectly) a maladaptive response.

SELF-CARE KNOWLEDGE: PERSONAL MODEL OF THE WORLD

Although humans have many perceptions in common, we each form our own unique perceptions of people, events, and situations. It is because each of us organizes and represents our experiences of people and things so differently that we nurses need to avoid jumping to conclusions about what people mean on the basis of their initial or surface comments to us. Most of us find this easy to understand when applied to abstractions such as justice, mercy, freedom, politics, and so forth. It is less often that we take into account our differences in cultures, subcultures, and life experiences that make one person's connotations of words such as *sick, well, easy, hard, frequently, seldom, hurt, pain, less, should*—even *always* and *never*—different from another's. "Depressed" can mean anything from a minor half-hour's alteration in mood to a severe debilitating state of inactivity and unconcern.

One person's pain may be another's challenge. Indeed, all of life events must be viewed from an individual's own perspective. What may seem like a minor occurrence to one may be a major catastrophe to another. An unanticipated pregnancy may be joy for one but agony for another. Weight loss may be perceived as positive for one and negative for another, or positive and negative for the same person at different times in that person's life. The way an individual perceives life, events, people, and situations, the way an individual communicates, thinks, feels, acts, and reacts—all of these factors—comprise the individual's *model of his or her world*. Each person's model is unique.

According to Milton Erickson, an appreciation for each individual's model of his or her world is a prerequisite for providing holistic care. Our understanding of the importance of this concept was acquired through the years by integrating Erickson's teachings with our experiences (11).

SUMMARY

We have described how nurses might consider individual uniqueness. We have said that people are different based on their inherent endowment, their current ability to mobilize resources needed to respond to stressors and distressors, and the way in which they model their world. Humans differ in important ways while simultaneously they are alike in other ways. These relationships are of importance to the nurse who provides holistic care.

NOTES

1. The word stressor was coined by Hans Selye as he developed his theory on stress and adaptation. His story is told in *The Stress of Life*, 2nd ed. (New York: McGraw-Hill, 1976).

2. This tendency to consider a single subsystem (wholism) rather than the holistic system seemed to result in different labels for similar (if not identical) phenomena.

3. Selye, *The Stress of Life*, p. 463. Hans Selye, *Stress Without Distress* (Philadelphia: Lippincott, 1974), pp. 28–29.

4. Walter Cannon, *The Wisdom of the Body*, rev. and enlarged ed. (New York: W. W. Norton & Co., Inc., 1963).

——, "Voodoo Death," *American Anthropologist* 44 (1942): 169–81. Arthur Schmale, "Relationship of Separation and Depression to Disease," *Psychosomatic Medicine* 20 (1958): 259–77. A. Schmale and H. Iker, "The Psychological Setting of Uterine Cervical Cancer," *Annals of New York Academy of Science* 125 (1966): 807–13.

5. G. Engel, *Psychological Development in Health and Disease* (Philadelphia: Saunders, 1962).

6. M. Seligman, *Helplessness* (San Francisco: W. H. Freeman & Company, Publishers, 1975).

7. Some nurses intuitively treat these individuals (those with potential for mobilizing resources and those without such potential) differently without knowing why. We hope this book will provide the theory for why such persons need different nursing care and for how to make such decisions in a more consistent and systematic fashion.

8. References for this work are: Helen Erickson, "Identification of States of Coping Utilizing Physiological and Psychosocial Data" (Master's thesis, The University of Michigan School of Nursing, 1976). Helen Erickson and Mary Ann Swain, "A Model for Assessing Potential Adaptation to Stress," *Research in Nursing and Health* 5, no. 2 (1982): pp. 93–101.

9. Selye, *Stress Without Distress*.

10. Richard Lazarus, *Psychological Stress and the Coping Process* (New York: McGraw-Hill, 1966).

11. Jeffrey Zeig, ed., *Ericksonian Approaches to Hypnosis and Psychotherapy* (New York: Brunner/Mazel, Inc., 1982).

Theoretical Formulations: The Linkages

OVERVIEW

In the preceding chapters we set forth our thoughts on how people are alike and how they differ. We presented several theorists for the reader to consider, each dealing with concepts that are important to nursing. Here we will describe the linkages among these concepts. While we have already implicitly alluded to many of these ideas, we would like to state them explicitly now. We hope that this integration will further assist you in understanding the potential impact of planned, goal-directed nursing interventions on the health and growth of the individual over time. We believe that our ideas about relationships among the concepts presented in the preceding chapters provide fertile ground for research activities. Our discussion in this chapter will focus on three central linkages: (1) the relationship between completion of developmental tasks and basic–need satisfaction, (2) the relationships among satisfaction of basic needs, object attachment and loss, and developmental growth, and (3) the relationship between one's ability to mobilize coping resources and need satisfaction.

DEVELOPMENTAL TASKS AND
BASIC-NEEDS SATISFACTION

We think that the degree to which developmental tasks are resolved is dependent on the degree to which human needs are satisfied. That is, as the individual encounters and works through the various developmental tasks of life, the outcome depends on the degree to which the basic needs are met. To help conceptualize these relationships, pause for a moment and think about building a home. Consider each developmental task as analogous to a part of the house. For example, the first stage of development (trust versus mistrust) is comparable to laying the foundation. The second stage (autonomy versus shame and doubt) could be compared to constructing the frame of the house; the third stage (initiative versus guilt) might be represented by the roof, and so forth. If, when you build your house, you use both effective and sufficient materials, you will most likely have a strong, well-constructed home when you're finished. But if, as you build your foundation, you fail to use sufficient cement, sand, water, and reinforcing wire, you will likely have a weak foundation. Although it might be strong enough to support the frame of the house, you may run into difficulty as you continue to build. Your foundation may begin to crack and possibly even crumble under the weight of additional parts of the house. The same goes for the frame, walls, and so forth. Finally, the house as a whole is only as durable as the sum of its parts, and each depends on the other for overall strength.

The satisfaction of basic needs at each step of development is as important as the use of good materials in the building of a house. Although most developmental tasks are more dependent on the satisfaction of some basic needs than are others, all tasks require that all basic needs be satisfied to a certain extent. The stage of trust requires that the physiological, safety-security, and belonging needs are well satisfied; the stage of industry is more dependent on satisfaction of the esteem and self–esteem needs than on physiological needs. In both stages, however, all basic needs emerge and must be satisfied.

More specifically, Erikson stated that during the first stage of life, people work through the task of developing trust. Maslow describes the basic (or survival) needs as physiological, safety-security, love-belonging, and esteem and self-esteem. Conceptually, then, putting the two together, as the mother responds to her infant's cries, body language, and verbalizations, she attempts to satisfy the infant's basic needs. If she is able to satisfy them *from the infant's perspective*, then the infant will gradually learn to have trust that his or her needs will be met. The outcome of task resolution will be a sense of trust with a pervading attitude of hope and a drive for the future.

We believe that these same relationships occur between the development of cognitive stages and the satisfaction of basic needs. For example, a four-year-old boy is exuberantly playing space war in the living room when his father comes home exhausted from a trying day at work. He ignores the child's greeting, settles into his chair, and opens the evening paper. The child continues to play at his feet, attempting to draw his father's attention to the game they have played together before. The father slams down the paper and yells at his son, "Go away. You're a pest." The father has threatened the boy's needs for safety, for belongingness, and for esteem. In addition, his actions interfere with the boy's developing ability to think in logical classes and to see relationships as others see them. His formerly acceptable behavior is relabeled as his being a "bad boy." His schemata about himself and his relationship to others are detrimentally impaired. If such interactive patterns are repeated, it is easy to see how there could be a subsequent relationship between cognitive and psychological growth. Children who have unmet basic needs have difficulty developing cognitively, which ultimately impacts on their psychological growth, and vice versa.

BASIC NEEDS, OBJECT ATTACHMENT AND LOSS, AND DEVELOPMENTAL GROWTH

There is also a linkage between object relationships and the satisfaction of human needs, such that object attachment is a vehicle for meeting basic needs. When an object repeatedly meets basic needs, attachment results. Thus, object loss results in basic-need deficits. A brief statement on how these notions apply to the experience of the infant may help clarify these relationships. At some point, the infant develops a sense of his or her primary care giver (usually the mother) as an object that provides comfort. The infant attaches to her as he or she experiences satisfaction of basic needs for food, warmth, comfort, safety, and affection. This happens as the mother responds to the infant's cries and other signals for attention. When her consistency and constancy are sufficient and the maturational time needed to internalize this experience has elapsed, the infant perceives the world as a basically trustworthy place and may be said to have completed the first developmental task.

Once the favorable ratio of basic trust to mistrust firmly exists, that same child, secure in the attachment to the care giver, risks trusting himself or herself to leave her intermittently to cruise out in exploration of an enlarging world and then runs back to the safety of the care giver's consistent availability after bumping up against new realities or problems to be solved, or simply to be refueled (1). Should the attachment figure prove untrustworthy at this time (that is, should the child sustain an object loss through some significant maternal inattentiveness or inability to continue nurturing and protecting), the child, perceiving rejection or abandonment, may either adopt a fearful overdependency, suppressing his or her own power to make reasonable choices, or an exaggerated independence that will not risk reliance on others. The child may "give up" self-control, rarely making significant decisions and rarely taking responsibility for them, or, conversely, the child may become highly invested in controlling all possible aspects of his or her life in a desperate attempt to feel safe and secure. The latter attitude especially may be coupled with a lack of concern for others. These results are indicative of a lack of autonomy.

We have noted that we cannot analyze data that clients present without discovering some form of object loss in connection with basic-need deficits. For example, feelings of insecurity are often associated with a sense of loss of permission for dependency due to the absence, withdrawal, or perceived distance of a significant other. If the loss occurred in the distant past, morbid grieving (2) and marked basic-need deficit coexist. It seems that in the course of life there are always some unresolved losses. The degree to which the lost objects were essential to need satisfaction determines the degree of morbid grieving that results. The greater the relationships between the lost object and the satisfaction of basic needs, the greater the deficit that occurs.

Consider, for example, the nine-month-old infant who is securely attached to mother. Loss of mother at this stage might well have a life-long impact. One case that comes to mind is that of a female client with diabetes, D., whose story is as follows:

> D. was the first child, born when her mother was 17 years old. When D. was 18 months old, a baby sister was born. The mother remained in the hospital for three weeks. During that time, D. was reported to have cried a lot, regressed in toilet training, and presented a general picture of misery. For comfort, she attached to a pillow. When the mother returned from the hospital she was busy with the new baby and fatigued from her difficulties. D. was now considered the big sister—too big to need to be helped, cuddled, and babied. D. clung to her pillow; it went everywhere with her, and eventually, of course, became very filthy! When she was four, D.'s father decided she was too old to carry "such a disgusting thing around." He took it from her and burned it. D. recalls the incident. From that time forth, she is described as having faked illness in order to get attention. Her mother said she would throw up, hold her breath, even lie down in the street hoping that a car would hit her. When she was eight, she was diagnosed as having juvenile onset diabetes. She has spent her life struggling with the conflicts associated with affiliated-individuation; now at the age of 32 she expresses the negative counterpart of all developmental tasks from trust through intimacy.

We think this client and her family would have benefited from holistic nursing care. The client had extensive basic-need deficits, evident from the time she experienced significant object loss in infancy. She had not constructively resolved any of the psychological developmental tasks; thus none of Erikson's virtues or strengths was evident. Both she and her family had spent years attempting to rework these early losses, never knowing how or why they were unsuccessful.

The degree to which needs are satisfied by object attachment depends on the availability of those objects and the degree to which they provide comfort and security as opposed to threat and anxiety. That is, a care giver might be the object of attachment but might not necessarily respond to the infant's request for need satisfaction in a way that would actually satisfy the infant's needs from the infant's perspective. If this should happen, there might be an anxious attachment instead of a secure attachment but, nevertheless, an attachment would develop. If this were the case, the infant might have a continuous sense of threatened safety-security or love-belonging. This state of affairs would ultimately interfere with the infant's ability to acquire a growth-producing balance of trust over mistrust.

Objects of importance vary across the life span. For example, small children derive comfort and love from very concrete objects, while healthy, older people tend to attach to more abstract, symbolic objects (such as a role, identity, a place, a thought, a relationship, or an ideal). Considering these differences across the life span helps the nurse in planning interventions. If some people have unresolved developmental tasks stemming from early childhood, the nurse might discover that the objects that take on significance for these persons are similar (though perhaps more sophisticated) to the objects that would have been expected in their earlier developmental stages. These individuals might surprise the nurse because these concrete, material objects seem even more important than interpersonal attachments, that is, objects more closely associated with the person's chronological age. As an example, a 35-year-old man may seem to be more interested in his motorcycle or car than he is in his family. It might help the nurse to clarify what his motorcycle represents by asking him what his "bike" means to him. She might discover that the only time he feels that he is in control (safe and secure) or feels important (self-esteem needs) is when he rides his bike!

Finally, if an individual seems to have had difficulty with an early developmental task, this might well provide a clue about the person's "favorite" way to conceptualize. These persons are not likely to be strong abstract thinkers, although they may have learned to think rather than to deal with their feelings (that is, they use intellectualization as a defense mechanism).

ADAPTIVE POTENTIAL
AND NEED SATISFACTION

By now it may seem apparent that an individual's potential for mobilizing resources—the person's state of coping according to the APAM—is directly associated with the person's need-satisfaction level. Individuals who have numerous basic-need deficits have limited potential for mobilizing self-care resources. These people are at great risk when they are confronted with stressors, whether ongoing or newly encountered. When nurses expect these people to learn new techniques in order to take care of themselves or comprehend information about a newly diagnosed illness, their self-care resources are further depleted. Such nursing interventions serve more as distressors than they serve to help the client attain a satisfactory state of health.

SUMMARY

As an individual works through the various developmental tasks of life, the degree to which that work results in a virtue and strength depends on the extent to which the basic needs are satisfied at each point. While some needs are more salient for some developmental tasks, all basic needs must be satisfied during the work on any developmental issue. The greater the basic-need deficits at any point in time, the less potential an individual has for mobilizing the resources needed to contend with new or ongoing stressors. Attachment to varying objects is the means by which individuals meet their needs. Early attachments are to concrete objects, but these attachments become increasingly abstract and symbolic in subsequent development. The implications of these relationships for nursing interventions will be discussed in Chapter 7.

NOTES

1. This is the process Mahler called separation-individuation.
2. Engel describes morbid grieving as a state in which the individual seems to be caught in a grief process. Behaviors vacillate between expressing angry feelings and engaging excessively in purposeless activities. G. L. Engel, "Grief and Grieving," *American Journal of Nursing* 64 (September 1964): 93.

Modeling and Role-Modeling: A Paradigm for Nursing Practice

OVERVIEW

In the preceding chapters we presented our philosophy, definition of nursing, theoretical bases from which we work, and our own theoretical statements about the relationships among these theory bases. We now describe our paradigm for the practice of professional nursing, emphasizing two major concepts: *modeling* and *role-modeling*. Since these terms have several connotations, we will be very specific about our definitions. We will describe each explicitly and then we will summarize the relationship between the two (1).

MODELING

The term *modeling* is often defined as the act of imitating a standard or copying a representation of something. The word *model* often refers to the standard or representation to be copied. In Chapter 5 we stated that each individual has a unique *model of his or her world*. One perceives one's environment from one's own perspectives, based on one's experiences, past learnings, state of life, and so forth. The act of modeling, then, is the process the nurse uses as she develops an image and understanding of the client's world—an image and understanding developed *within the client's framework and from the client's perspective.*

Modeling contains the art and the science of nursing. That is, the *art of modeling* is the development of a mirror image of the situation from the client's perspective. It requires communication skills basic to nursing. These skills will help the nurse put one foot into a word foreign to herself. The *science of modeling* is the scientific aggregation and analysis of the data collected about the *client's model.* The science of modeling requires keeping the other foot firmly planted in the theoretical bases discussed above.

ROLE-MODELING

Role-modeling cannot occur until the nurse has modeled her *client's world* and has aggregated and analyzed the constructs of that world. Role-modeling is the facilitation of the individual in attaining, maintaining, or promoting health through purposeful interventions. These interventions are planned based on the data analyses.

Role-modeling is also both an art and a science. The *art of role-modeling* occurs when the nurse plans and implements interventions that are unique for her client. The *science of role-modeling* occurs as the nurse plans interventions with respect to her theoretical base for the practice of nursing. For example, a client might have basic unmet security needs and be working on the stage of autonomy. Scientifically, the nurse would plan interventions that would promote perceived trust and control, but these interventions would have to be designed based on the individual's personal perceptions and beliefs—*the individual's model of the world.*

Role-modeling is, in our minds, the essence of nurturance. It is the basis for the predictive and prescriptive component of nursing practice. Role-modeling requires an unconditional acceptance of the person as the person is while gently encouraging and facilitating growth and development at the person's own pace and *within the person's own model.*

MODELING AND ROLE-MODELING

One author had a client whose developmental history resulted in nonresolution of all of the developmental tasks. Her basic-need deficits were multiple and severe; she had experienced those deficits throughout her 28 years. Her recurrent mode of trying to satisfy those basic needs (*modeling*) was to alternate between showering others with gifts ("I don't need anything. I'll give to you") and becoming gravely ill, necessitating hospitalization ("You take complete care of me"). Her basic-need deficits were seen graphically in her inability to identify any personal strengths. In an attempt to move this client toward a healthier state, the nurse gave this client gifts of her strengths (*role-modeling*). That is, the nurse wrote down strengths she had identified in this client, wrapped them attractively, and presented them as gifts (2).

We have found it preeminently important to enter for a time into our *client's world*, to share as empathetically as we can *the client's model* of it. As we work from within *that model*—in a true partnership with our client—we are better able to support adaptive coping and suggest strategies that are acceptable to both nurse and client. *Modeling* occurs as the nurse accepts and understands her client; *role-modeling* starts the second the nurse moves from the analysis phase of the nursing process to the planning of nursing interventions.

Because each one has a *personal model of the world*, people with nursing needs are not helped in standardized ways. We do not have it within ourselves to know how a unique individual may best be helped; only the individual knows the kind of help he or she needs to mobilize strengths and resources. At some level, people know what has made them sick or distressed, and they know what will make them well or help them feel better. If people do not know this consciously, a skillful nurse can help them learn to know and express themselves, thus identifying the particular assistance they want and need. It is in this context that our concept of self-care has taken shape. For us, self-care is not merely a choice of options within a framework chosen for a patient or designated by the nurse or other professional. We believe self-care for health is broader than that. Our experiences in nursing have convinced us that people have more control and responsibility over their health than they (or their care providers) often realize. They will take that control when they are permitted, invited, and patiently encouraged to do so. In the long run, the one person best equipped to remain in charge and ultimately accountable for goal setting and coordination of his or her own health care is the consumer who contracts for help.

When we refer to the responsibility people have for their health care, it is not our intention to assign blame for deviations from desired states of comfort and function. Rather, since each person has a *unique model*—a specific way of getting basic needs met—each person also has the key to what he or she personally needs.

People also know best their individual timing for change. As they live in families and societies that are inevitably affected by changes in one member, they may move toward change more slowly than we might desire. It frees us from assuming inordinate responsibility to remember that, however great our concern and good will for our clients, making a decision to change is ultimately their prerogative and should be done according to their timeline. Indisputably, they have control over such decisions and we always keep this in mind. We can extend genuine invitations to live and to live well, while standing by without rejecting or abandoning our clients. While waiting and unconditionally accepting them, we continue to facilitate and nurture their growth and development. Nurses interested in providing holistic care will find that *modeling* and *role-modeling* will give them freedom to help their clients explore and utilize many alternative means to attaining, promoting, and maintaining health. There are more ways than one to relax, lose weight, reduce pain, fight infection, heal wounds, walk again, "get better," and so forth.

SUMMARY

Our paradigm for the practice of professional nursing integrates *modeling* and *role-modeling*. *Modeling* is the process by which the nurse seeking to understand her client's unique model of the world. *Role-modeling* is the process by which the nurse understands that unique model within the context of scientific theories and, using that same perspective of her client's unique model, plans interventions that promote health. In Part III we will deal with how these concepts are applied in the nursing process.

NOTES

1. The initial formulation of *modeling* and *role–modeling* was first articulated for us by Milton H. Erickson, M.D., a master in operationalizing both concepts. We feel deeply indebted to him for many important learnings related to these ideas. His work has been an inspiration and provided us with direction. You might enjoy reading his work. Although there are many things he has written that would be of assistance, we recommend that you start with *Uncommon Therapy: The Teachings of Milton Erickson* by Jay Haley (New York: W. W. Norton & Co., Inc., 1973).

2. This client had been hospitalized for more than 300 days the year before the nurse began working with her. The three years before that she had spent from 200 to 300 days per year in the hospital. She was on social security disability, had not had a job for more than five years, and was unable to function independently when she began working with the nurse four and one-half years ago. At the time of this writing she has been hospitalized fewer than 100 days in four and one-half years, has returned to work, is off social security disability, has moved to another state, and is functioning independently. She still calls her nurse when emergencies arise (about every four to six months). From her perspective, the nurse–client relationship has "saved her life." When she is asked what the nurse does for her, she comments that the nurse "cares about her," accepts her as she is, and has helped her to "become."

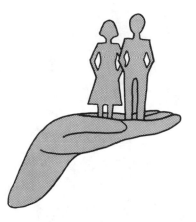

III

MODELING AND ROLE-MODELING: PRACTICAL CONSIDERATIONS

In Part II we presented our theory and paradigm for nursing, including the functional relationships among the concepts. In Part III we will present practical considerations for implementing these ideas. Using a nursing paradigm that incorporates modeling the client's world before and during the planning of interventions requires a flexible, creative nurse. It would be so simple if we could standardize interventions with formulas, such as "Basic love-need deficit: give five hugs daily!" Unfortunately, it isn't that simple. Role–modeling requires that we step into the client's world before we plan interventions. Take, for example, the client who had had a myocardial infarction who couldn't seem to recover until he got a dog. He then made a remarkable recovery. Certainly, his dog met several basic needs, and by now, you can probably name which ones, and how the dog met them. We all know that this man's solution does not mean that all postinfarct clients should be encouraged to get a dog. Some people don't like dogs. However, for this man, a dog symbolized many things, all related to basic-need satisfaction, and was therefore an important intervention.

Designing interventions that truly help people requires that a nursing process take place. The paradigm laid out in the preceding pages suggests that the nurse need not use a straightforward, cut-and-dried approach while making nursing diagnoses and planning care. At the same time, we urge you to be systematic, keeping your mind immersed and anchored in the theory bases that you are using. This, of course, is not a simple thing to do. Some would say, "How do you keep *head and heart in gear at the same time?" Our only response is that it takes practice and courage, but over time it becomes as comfortable as an old shoe. Part III will help you organize your thinking so that you can learn how to implement our ideas. It is organized around the following major themes:*

Nursing process: general considerations
How does one collect data?
How does one aggregate, analyze, and synthesize data?
What does one think about while planning interventions?
What personal characteristics does one need to use the paradigm?

8

Nursing Process

The term *nursing process* is currently used by nurses in two distinct, yet related ways. Perhaps most commonly, the expression represents nursing's special terminology for simple problem solving, a formal, ordered process that includes collecting and analyzing data, suggesting possible solutions, implementing them, evaluating outcomes, and restarting the entire cycle as needed.

A second and more basic use of the term refers to the ongoing, interactive exchange of information, feelings, and behavior between the nurse and client(s), wherein the nurse's goal is to nurture and support the client's self-care. Our emphasis on modeling and role-modeling refocuses attention on the importance of the interactive, interpersonal nursing process.

In this chapter we will briefly discuss how we view the relationship between the two current connotations of nursing process and describe some practical implications of our emphasis on the interactive nurse–client relationship in giving holistic care.

INTERACTIVE NURSING PROCESS
IS PRIMARY

We value a reemphasis on the primacy of the interactive, interpersonal nature of the nursing process. In our zeal to establish nursing on a firm scientific foundation, some of us have lost sight of this broader, historically earlier, and more fundamental connotation of nursing process as the ongoing, interactive exchange that occurs when a caring, competent nurse relates to a client to nurture and support the client's growth and development toward health (1).

We agree with Kinlein that nursing care begins from the moment of contact (2). Every practicing nurse vividly recalls clients initially contacted in acute care situations who expressed high anxiety in both word and body. These people need immediate nursing intervention that cannot wait for a formal nursing interview (3). In order to even begin expressing their real needs, most people need the holistic skills of a nurse who enters into an interpersonal relationship with them. The nurse's first and primary contribution to such clients is her whole self—her presence, acceptance, and comfort-promoting skill expressed in both concrete and symbolic ways (4). Whether inside institutions or out, expert nursing facilitates a client's expression of what brings the client for care and helps the client discover *what he or she already knows* that will help him or her feel better or achieve optimum health.

Underlying and supporting an effective nurse–client relationship are the theoretical bases and skills developed by systematically practicing scientific habits of thought. Scientific habits of thought are not unique to nursing. What is unique, and very special, is a holistic interactive, interpersonal relationship between the nurse and client.

Often when nurses use the term nursing process, they think first of an ordered set of operations by which they collect and analyze a particular sequence and quantity of data from a predetermined group of categories and then identify problems that they and their *patients* solve "together" (5). In our opinion, this connotation of the term has led many nurses to view the nursing process as a cumbersome task to be completed. Some have come to believe that they must focus on maintaining a routine, step-by-step sequence, collecting comprehensive amounts of data, identifying all of a patient's problems

before they can initiate any nursing care. We have directly contra-
dicted this notion by stating that nursing care begins from the first
moment of client contact. By emphasizing a method and prespecified
content, this view favors the formalized nursing process over the interactive, interpersonal process that is so central to nursing.

We do not therefore usually follow a rigid sequence, wherein
we first collect all data, sit down to analyze it, plan each intervention
in advance, then intervene, and finally evaluate. We think this is
neither needed nor practical in many situations. A nurse rolls up her
sleeves from the first moment of contact, *intervening* from the start,
by *listening* while analyzing and evaluating; *analyzing* while listening, intervening, and evaluating; *evaluating* while intervening,
analyzing, and listening—in short, doing the nursing process (as
general problem solving) in her head while simultaneously giving
care. We can hardly emphasize enough that, in order to engage skillfully in a purposive, on-the-spot therapeutic process, a nurse needs
to internalize a comprehensive framework or paradigm for giving
care.

We are saying that nurses can feel comfortable even if a comprehensive formal data collection is not treated as a priority. They
can be confident that much effective nursing occurs before any bit
of data is ever formally collected, analyzed, and recorded. Nevertheless, we value the formal aspect of the nursing process because we
believe that there are important scientific and therapeutic habits to
be developed. Skilled nursing practitioners who have internalized
these habits of thought can collapse and vary the process as we have
described above (6).

When we view the nursing process predominantly as an ongoing, interactive, interpersonal relationship that *includes* use of the
formal scientific mode of thought, we can regard documentation of
the nursing process primarily as a valuable way to communicate
with others and keep records. Primary and consulting nurses find
that systematic, clear recordings serve to convey to colleagues a rationale for their recommendations. This has particular benefit when
it promotes consistency in the nursing care given by other nurse
members on the team. Naturally, too, careful documentation helps
us formulate questions for nursing research, enabling us to compare
and contrast our clients' experiences.

There are times when we have found it useful to assess, analyze,
diagnose, and plan in that precise order. In particularly complex or

frustrating nursing care situations, the time and effort taken to record data and then ponder it has resulted in insights not so immediately apparent during the actual moments of client contact.

IMPLICATIONS OF OUR VIEW
OF THE NURSING PROCESS

Expressed Needs Direct
the Physical Assessment

Because we always start *where the client is* (*modeling*), inviting full
and free expression of worries, questions, or concerns, we rarely do
"routine" comprehensive assessments during which *we* direct the
content, sequence and amount of information gathered. This is particularly true of the assessment of the biophysical subsystem and its
related physical statuses or body systems.

Unless the client personally asks for a comprehensive, all subsystem, all statuses within subsystems, assessment as a result of the
nursing care we give, we do not waste our time routinely collecting
and recording arbitrary amounts of data not needed to achieve nursing goals. Tiring or boring clients by lengthy biophysical examinations already done by a physician conflicts with the prior nursing
principle of reducing a person's stressors. Duplicating the work of
physicians is wasteful; it also robs clients of time and energy. We
rely on what the physician has done. Thus, we think *comprehensive*
physical assessments done by nurses are only infrequently needed
to deliver good nursing care. *Impoverished* persons and clients who
want help in special disease-preventive and health-enhancement
contexts provide exceptions (7).

If the *client* indicates a concern or need for help in relation to a
particular physical status, the client may be asked or invited to share
additional detail, and a physical examination of a specific part may
follow. This is done in as much detail and incorporates as many related statuses or body systems as the nurse judges necessary to promote the person's optimum self-care. The particular nature, depth,
and breadth of investigation develop in synchrony with continued
input from the client whom we invariably invite and encourage to
participate *with* us in the examination. This is done through, among

other things, sharing our immediate findings in a natural, sensitive, and nonthreatening way (8).

Below is an example in which this approach facilitated a client's holistic self-care. Her identified reason for coming for care was to consult one of us about her recurrent breast lumps.

> The client had undergone repeated negative biopsies. Now her concern to detect any possible cancer early began clashing with fears of potentially endless future biopsies. On her arrival at the office, she was invited to begin *wherever she wished to start*. While the nurse actively listened, the client began talking about current family tensions and did not mention the lumps again until a half-hour later when she asked the nurse to feel the lump that was currently worrying her so. The nurse gently palpated a one-by-two centimeter oval lump while verbalizing her findings in simple, descriptive ways. She placed the client's hand on the breast to enable the client to feel for herself what the nurse had described. A moment later when the client commented, "I feel so relaxed with you" (and looked it), the nurse immediately reexamined the lump (without any change in the client's position) and found it gone. The client's hand was guided back without comment, allowing her to note that phenomenon for herself. Integrating her two self-examinations with her own last comment and the earlier discussion about her family, the client drew her own conclusion—slowly and thoughtfully—and then said, "Is it possible that my tensions are responsible for some of the scary signs I've been getting over and over again? I *do* know that I'm more aware of the lump when I'm upset!" (9).

The example illustrates once more that dynamic holism wherein psychic concerns have physiological influences, and vice versa. It principally highlights how the nurse's response while using a theory-based paradigm for giving care to a whole person facilitates a quality of self-care and self-discovering not possible with a linear nursing model (10).

We want our views about this subject to be very clear. We strongly believe that nurses need to know *how* to collect a full range of data in each of the subsystems (biophysical, psychological, social, cognitive) and how to aggregate that information within the context of our current understanding of normal functioning. *Whether* the nurse collects it—and how much the nurse collects from and within each subsystem—always related to the expressed needs and desires of the client. For example, when a client wants help with a physical concern, such as engaging relief measures for labored breathing, or learning to live with chronic shortness of breath, we need to gather the data important to establish a base line that we will *share* in order to implement *together* relief measures that are safe for the client, and also to monitor *with the client* the improvements we observe over time. There are situations in which we do collect biophysical data in the absence of the client's direction to do so. In intensive care situations, in which individuals are often *impoverished,* we naturally establish immediate biophysical base lines for our anticipated periodic exchanges with these clients. Our intensive care clients have much more easily accepted, even embraced, their medical recommendations for fluid restrictions when by mutual agreement they were regularly informed of fluid levels in their lungs.

Client Concerns Preempt
Nurse-Identified Problems

We have virtually abandoned the problem-oriented approach within this paradigm. This approach implies that nurses objectively know what *patients* need and that they can decide, based on their expertise, what is best for *patients*. In other words, we view the notion of a nurse-identified problem as being contrary to our view that the *client* knows best what contributed to the illness and what will make the client better.

When nurses identify problems that have no current relevance to the client's expressed concerns, their efforts to develop plans and intervene with these persons are often ineffective. They become frustrated trying to implement interventions for diagnoses that have priority only for members of the health care team. Documentation, if done, dissolves into uninspiring busy work that provides little insight or assistance to colleagues. Persons whose real, immediate concerns are unattended do not progress as the nurses expect. Faced with the need to assist numerous clients concurrently and working without a unifying theory base, nurses tend to substitute cursory material for the all-inclusive, problem-oriented recordings they once learned to write. Some keep struggling all the while for the time and opportunity to do something they call "the nursing process." We want to encourage staff nurses to put aside their false guilts and begin to experience a theory-based interactive, interpersonal process with clients that can lead to satisfying, effective nursing care that incorporates subsequent documentation of *significant* nursing (not medical) observations—nursing (not medical) goals, means, and progress.

Our experience with clients who have multiple health concerns has been that when we begin with the client's most immediate concern and help the client with what is most important to the client, one of two things happens: Either a gradual successive uncovering of significant unmet needs occurs or the client, himself or herself, takes care of many of his or her remaining unmet needs as a natural consequence of their dynamic interrelatedness and the inherent drive toward health. Because of the person's holistic nature, if the person resolves one concern, that healthier state impacts on other aspects of his or her total being. An illustration follows:

A woman in her sixties was being treated medically with radiation and chemotherapy following surgery for removal of a cancer that had subsequently spread widely throughout her body. Her physicians judged that she was not responding to their current treatment as they had expected.

Her white blood count and resistance to infection were dangerously low. She had no appetite, had developed pneumonia, and was plagued with intense pain on moving in bed, especially when getting out of bed to attend to toileting needs. She requested help from the nurse. She wanted to talk about preparing herself for what her doctors had concluded would be her soon and certain death.

When first seen by the nurse, the woman complained of deep fatigue. Her color was gray. She was short of breath, was lying stiffly in bed, had lines in her forehead, and had lackluster eyes. She spoke slowly and softly with many short sighs interspersed.

As the nurse sat beside her bed ready to carry out their explicit contract to deal with her concern about dying, the nurse noted that her client ranged in random fashion from topic to topic, none of which touched on the subject of dying. She spoke of her extreme weakness and fatigue, of her sadness seeing her husband's emotional response to her deteriorating condition, of the excruciating nature of her pain when getting out of bed, her terror of its inevitable recurrence because the alternative of using a bedpan was "even worse." She lamented her inability to believe her doctors when they spoke of their findings and their earlier expressed hope for her favorable response to therapy. She felt exhausted from her visitors but would not ask any of them to shorten their stays or postpone their visits. She would sacrifice any mention of her particular wants or needs to a preeminent need to be liked and approved by the nurses as an undemanding "good patient." She would say, "There are others on the unit who need the nurses' care more than I."

She had spent precious energy giving gifts to and "entertaining" many of the nurses who with genuine personal affection and sympathy frequently stopped by her bedside to say a cheery word to this "incredible lady" who had so many friends and whose condition and prognosis were so "hopeless and tragic."

After establishing through active listening that the patient's main concern *now* was her pain on getting up out of bed, the nurse contracted to set a time together to exchange information, feelings, knowledge, and skills in an effort to find a way to work with or reduce that pain to a tolerable level. Setting this simple goal in itself required much reassurance of the nurse's willingness to spend the necessary effort to carry out the plan. Mrs. A suffered a severe loss of self-esteem and found it hard to believe that she could be "worth so much time and attention." Hesitantly, she gave the nurse the very essential data she, alone, knew about her past efforts and experiences during attempts to get up.

The 15 minutes spent working together on this problem required continuous attention to Mrs. A's sense of safety and security: her fear of encountering a pain over which she would have no control, her repeatedly verbalized reluctance to bother the busy nurse by taking her time in this manner. At first, she believed herself helpless and lacking the ability to make any contribution to the project—even discounting the usefulness of describing her anticipated fears and present-moment sensations—until she was reassured by a variety of means, including gentle, yet confident voice tones, thoughtfully placed touches, soft smiles, and a bit of humor.

The time the nurse took to deal with Mrs. A's escalated fear, and the control the nurse repeatedly gave back to her over the "what if's" she raised, finally paid off. As Mrs. A chose from the nurse's suggestions those that she felt she could handle, she built on each successful step of an incremental process to bring herself to a sitting position on the side of the bed entirely on her own power.

Sitting on the side of the bed, shaking her head in disbelief at having raised herself up without a twinge of pain, she gave a deep sigh of relief and said, "For the first time I have hope!" She promptly launched into an animated description of how she would now be able to get up to the bathroom freely where she would assume "the only sitting position" that would enable her to deep breathe and cough without aggravating her pain. Although she knew how important deep breathing was to combat the pneumonia, she had been falsely reporting to the nurses her compliance with these doctor's "orders" because of the extreme pain and her fear of displeasing her care givers. She also volunteered that she had been limiting her own fluid intake to reduce the number of times she needed to get up out of bed but would no longer risk giving herself a urinary tract infection through that practice. She requested a favorite sandwich for dinner, affirming that she knew she would be able to "keep it down" now. And she capped her remarks by announcing her intention to live at least " 'til Christmas" (six months away) to fulfill a special dream she had earlier abandoned.

She did indeed follow through on every one of her own decisions. Within a few days, she amazed her physicians who asked her, "Just what did that nurse do to 'turn you around'?" She laughed merrily when she reported that they wanted to learn the particular method by which she had brought herself up to the side of the bed. She herself knew that, while she had indeed taken advantage of some important principles of body mechanics, what had really happened was a reactivation and resumption of her self-care actions through an integrative nursing process that had restored her hope and belief in herself as a worthwhile person. She herself had accepted the nurse's invitation to actively take her strengths and the power she still had— to choose to live!

Having said all that we have about comprehensive, formal, problem-oriented approaches to the nursing process, you may wonder why we structured the following chapters in a traditional format. We know people need to be able to incorporate new knowledge into their existing cognitive framework if that knowledge is to be useful. Therefore, in order to help you assimilate and accommodate knowledge, we have ordered our thoughts in that way.

Our dissatisfaction is not with the formal scientific process itself, but with the manner in which that formal process has been interpreted. Our objections are threefold:

1. The interactive, interpersonal nature of the process has not been emphasized enough.
2. The overemphasis on comprehensiveness and problem solving tends to ignore the *client's model of his or her world* and the client's strengths.
3. The emphasis on systematic documentation first is unrealistic in many situations because it frustrates busy nurses who could be giving scientific care.

We accept as legitimate the steps of a scientific therapeutic process. In the next chapters we discuss that formal nursing process in detail from the perspective of the modeling and role-modeling paradigm. Because the formal aspect occurs within the interactive, interpersonal aspect of the nursing process, there is still much room for flexibility and creativity of format in organizing our ideas. We have yet to learn all the "best" ways of communicating nursing principles and practices to one another.

SUMMARY

Dual use of the term nursing process exists. The term is used for formal problem solving and for the more basic interactive, interpersonal process that nurtures and supports the person's self-care. Students and graduates of nursing have met such heavy requirements for written work that some have lost sight of the way that the *problem-solving nursing process* slots into the larger concept of the *interactive nursing process*. Detailed paperwork that contains a multitude of nurse-identified problems is a poor substitute for one or more key nursing diagnoses that relate to the client's primary concerns. When nurses experience the nursing process as the lively, significant, and productive interaction between nurse and client—whether or not *problem* identification by the client occurs—they will gather and record data that are truly relevant to achievable mutual goals. They will communicate clearly with colleagues to the ultimate benefit of clients and their own personal and professional satisfaction.

NOTES

1. Consider the following quotations from Hildegard Peplau, *Interpersonal Relations in Nursing* (New York: Putnam's, 1952).

Nursing is a significant, therapeutic interpersonal process. (p. 16)

Interpersonal interactions between a patient and nurse—either as a person recognized in her own right or as a personification of an earlier figure in the patient's life—are often more telling in the outcome of a patient's problem than are many routine technical procedures. (p. 6)

For purposes of nursing practice, a personal relationship is one in which two persons come to know one another well enough to face the problem at hand in a co-operative way. (p. 9)

. . . the interpersonal nursing process is therapeutic when needs are met in a way that refreshes and restores the patient for meeting new problems. (p. 9)

2. Lucille Kinlein, *Independent Nursing Practice with Clients* (Philadelphia: Lippincott, 1977), p. 61. We authors have noted that student nurses who are explicitly told they cannot give nursing care until they have collected information, analyzed it, identified a "problem," and preplanned their nursing actions easily conclude that the "nursing process" is a *task* that becomes an end in itself, rather than a description of what is present in an open, honest, warm exchange between two holistic persons, the nurse and her client. Similarly, we have heard staff nurses bemoan a lack of time to "do" the nursing process. This suggests they are focusing on a formal set of operations, usually "problem-oriented," requiring a measurable block of time for its completion. They seem to be saying that because time for "the nursing process" has not been written into their contracts with their employing institutions, they are prevented from practicing quality nursing.

3. Clients first seen on admission to an overnight unit in a hospital are often in a state of *impoverishment* from having spent energy in admitting or emergency rooms or from having already given a physician whatever data help to initiate earliest medical relief measures.

4. *Therapeutic use of self* has a long history in the nursing literature. See Peplau's statement from p. 16 in note 1 above.

5. This particular description of a nursing process, although very common, conflicts with our paradigm because the nurse pre-determines the sequence, quantity, and categories of data collection. The nurse, then identifies "problems" that the person (who is being treated as a *patient*) should solve. Many nurses give lip service to solving problems *with* a person, but our experience suggests that although the patient's input is solicited about possible solutions, the patient is rarely consulted for his or her view as to whether the nurse-identified problem really is a *problem* to *him or her.*

6. See *Nursing: A Social Policy Statement*, American Nurses Association, 1980, pp. 12–13.

7. Some might object to the expression "health enhancement," given a definition of health as optimum bio-psycho-socio-spiritual function. One of us uses the expression to refer to clients who to all observers may be functioning at a high level of health and yet desire help reaching an ever-higher potential in their growth and development.

8. Sensitive, nonthreatening sharing presupposes effective prior *modeling* of the *client's world.*

9. At the time of this contact, we could not assertively confirm a relationship between breast lumps and psychic tension because we knew of no controlled studies establishing correlation between breast changes of this kind and subjective feeling states. We believe experiences in nursing processes of this kind can become more common for nurses and will become the substance from which a nursing science of *health* will continue to develop. We think we have not yet begun to tape and organize the vast fund of information buried in the minds, hearts, and experiences of effective nurses (and their clients) about the normal, healthy functioning of ever-changing holistic persons. We have yet to hypothesize, test, and formulate scientific principles of health and health care that so naturally fall within professional nursing's range of concern.

Question: At this point in her life experience, did this client's fear of cancer plus potentially endless biopsies combine to create body changes associated with neuro-humoral secretion and related fluid shifts? In what way might her experience of current "tensions" within the family contribute to any physiological effects?

Question: If clients receive holistic nursing, will they make and integrate sufficiently significant observations about themselves to prevent procedures such as bilateral prophylactic mastectomies from ever becoming a tragic echo of myriad past hysterectomies now openly acknowledged to have been unnecessary?

10. Linear models partake of single relationships: causative or correlative. The medical model has been sometimes called a *linear model*.

How Does One Collect Data?

OVERVIEW

In Chapter 8 we provided an overview for the remaining chapters in Part III. We stated that each chapter would address a step in the nursing process. Our purpose in this chapter is to help you organize your thoughts as you collect data. Specifically, we will help you address the following questions: Where shall I get my data? How should I systematically collect it?

DATA SOURCES

You will want to remember two things as you seek data. First, your goal is to develop an interactive, interpersonal working relationship with your client that will assist the client to attain and maintain optimum health given the circumstances. Second, you have several sources of information, but your *primary and most important source is your client*. Without the client's input you will be unable to understand which nursing interventions are clearly needed.

If your client is comatose and unable to communicate verbally,

you will need to rely more heavily on the secondary sources of information. At this time, you will place heavy emphasis on the data
provided by family and friends while continuing to focus on the
client's self-care. You will remember that even comatose persons
have strengths. Their strengths may be as simple as the functioning
of the heart, lungs, or brain; nevertheless, these are strengths.

While your primary source of data is your client, your secondary sources are (1) the nurse's observations and (2) the client's friends
and family. You and your nurse colleagues are important sources of
data. You will make observations that are important in the person's
total care. Specifically, these observations might include physical
data, observations of family interactions, progress toward desired
goals, client's verbal and nonverbal actions, client's response to you,
and so forth.

Sometimes you will be unable to collect data from family and
friends. Nevertheless, since people strive toward affiliated-individuation, it is necessary for you to try. At times it may mean that you
will have to call long distance or arrange to meet these people off-
duty. Since your first intent is to develop an interactive, interpersonal relationship with your client, remember to include the client
in the decision to talk with the family whenever possible. Whenever
possible, data collection from family sources is done in the presence
of your client. At a minimum, you will want to provide the client
with feedback on the process. You may wonder when it is necessary
for you to collect information from the family. There are several situations in which this is helpful. A few examples are when your client
is unable to speak (comatose), when your client requests that you
speak with the family, when you think there are important data family members can provide about your client that the client is unable
to provide, and when the family members wish to speak with you.

The tertiary sources of data include the medical care team and
other health care team members. Sometimes you will want (and
need) information from the physician concerning his or her assessment, diagnosis, and medical care plan. This is particularly important when you are trying to assist an individual to attain health. The
more important the sickness problem is to the client, the more likely
you will want this information. The other members of the health
care team also contribute tertiary data. Sometimes they will be involved in the care of your client and you will want to know what
they are saying, planning, and doing. These professionals include
dieticians, physical therapists, respiratory therapists, social work-

ers, and so forth. Sometimes the doctor will request their assistance, and at other times you will request it. In either case, these people will often provide you with important information needed to provide holistic nursing care.

Thus far we have said that there are three major sources:

1. The client
2. The nurse
   The family and friends
3. The medical team's observations and plans
   Other health care team members' observations and plans

The first is your primary source of data; the next two constitute your secondary sources of data; the last two are your tertiary sources of data. You will use your professional judgment to determine when you need to seek the tertiary sources of information. You will always seek the primary source first and then the secondary source. Your care will be planned based on an aggregation of the data obtained from these sources.

DATA ORGANIZATION

We will now consider the *kinds* of data that need to be collected and how to organize them. We believe that there are four major categories you can use to structure this process:

1. Description of the situation
2. Expectations
3. Resource potential
4. Goals and life tasks

The purpose for data collection within each of these major categories is to be able to interpret the data and specify nursing diagnoses. Each category also has subcategories for data collection. Each subcategory assists the nurse to specify the data in terms of the purpose for collecting data. Table 9-1 shows the categories, subcategories, and purposes for data collection. Table 9-2 provides a format for data collection, including all three sources of information

TABLE 9-1 Categories, Subcategories, and Purposes
for Data Collection

Category and Subcategories	Purpose of Data Collection
Description of the Situation	
1. Overview of the situation	1. To develop an overview of the client's situation from the client's perspective

2. Etiology
    Stressors
    Distressors
	2. To identify the etiological factors involved

3. Therapeutic needs	3. To identify possible therapeutic interventions
Expectations	
1. Immediate	1. To develop an understanding of the client's personal orientation in terms of the client's expectation for the present and future
2. Long-term	
Resource Potential	

1. External
    Social network
    Support system
    Health care system
	1. To determine the nature of the external support system

2. Internal
    Strengths
    Adaptive potential
    Feeling states
    Physiological data
	2. (a) To determine the client's strengths and virtues
	   (b) To determine the client's currently available internal resources

Goals and Life Tasks	
1. Current 2. Future	1. To determine the current developmental status in order to understand the client's personal model and to utilize maximum communication skills

plus categories and subcategories of data. We remind you that we don't believe you need to collect data from all sources before you start interventions, but you do need to begin with your client's self-care knowledge whenever possible. The remainder of this chapter is organized in terms of the three sources of information with details about data to be collected from each category and subcategory.

TABLE 9-2 Data Collection Format with Three Sources of Data

Data Categories	Primary Self-care Knowledge	Secondary		Tertiary*	
		Nurse's Observations	Family, Friends' Observations	Physician's Observations and Plans	Others' Observations and Plans
Description of the Situation					
1. Overview of the situation					
2. Etiology					
Stressors					
Distressors					
3. Therapeutic Needs					
Expectations					
1. Immediate					
2. Long-term					
Resource Potential					
1. External					
Social network					
Support system					
Health care system					
2. Internal					
Strengths					
Adaptive Potential					
Feeling states					
Physiological data					
Goals and Life Tasks					
1. Current					
2. Future					

*You will include the medical diagnosis, etiological factors, plans, and expectations in this column.

SELF-CARE KNOWLEDGE

Description of the Situation

You need to ascertain your client's description of the situation in order to determine what factors the client perceives as stressors precipitating or amplifying the current situation. You may also identify some stressors that your client doesn't name, or you might even make some guesses after you hear the client's story. However, you'll need to ask the client how he or she feels about your perspectives before you determine whether or not they are really issues for further consideration. Let's take, for example, the 55-year-old male who is admitted with acute chest pain. He may say that the problem was precipitated by what he ate for dinner, and then tell you that he and his wife had spent the evening chatting, except for a short time when he received a phone call. If you ask him to elaborate on what he and his wife talked about, he might say that they were discussing their budget or if you ask about the telephone call he might say that his boss had called about a meeting the following day. You might conclude that there *may* have been more to the evening than pleasant, non-stressful events. The evening might have been riddled with distressors, *but you will not know what he really thinks unless you ask your client*. The only thing for sure is that at the moment he is saying that it was his dinner, so you'd probably benefit from respecting that perspective, since your client is probably *impoverished* (1) at this time. Nevertheless, you will keep in mind that there might be many distressors not yet identified.

In most cases, however, individuals can explicitly describe what they perceive as the problem. For example:

> There was the woman who visited the cardiologist to be treated for angina and palpitations. The physician found no organic medical problem and therefore turned to the nurse for assistance. When the nurse asked what was causing the problem the woman stated very simply, "My husband died two weeks ago." The nurse, familiar with the theoretical bases presented in Chapters 4 and 5, had no difficulty in understanding the importance of this statement and planning interventions that would help this woman adapt to the loss of her husband.

You will also ask your client what he or she thinks will make him or her feel better. People have interesting ideas about what makes them sick—and what will make them well. Most of the time these remedies are symbolic of something else (just as the dog in an earlier example), but it doesn't matter what their remedy symbolizes so long as it does the trick. How many times have we ourselves said such things as "a dish of ice cream would sure make me feel better," or "I feel better just getting it off my chest." We health care providers often assume that we know what will help, but we don't take into account that we're talking and thinking from our own perspective. Sometimes something that helps one will also help another and sometimes it won't.

We have had clients who have said that what they need is just to come to talk to us and they will get better. The woman described above who had just lost her husband was such an example. There are many others too. Consider the hypertensive client who discovered that all he needed to do to get his blood pressure to come down to a normal reading was to pick up the telephone to call his nurse. This person later learned (with purposeful interventions) (2) that he didn't even need to call. He could just "think" what the conversations would be about, and that would bring his blood pressure down. Or take as another example the small child who is experiencing separation-individuation anxiety when mommy goes off to work (3). When asked what will make him feel better, he might say, "To have mommy with me." Why not give him mommy, then? That is, why not give him mommy in a symbolic yet concrete way. A picture of mom, tucked neatly into a pocket or pinned to his undershirt, somewhere he can *feel* it, will often relieve such anxiety and facilitate this small child's march out into the big, scary world.

We have said that we need to collect data from our client's perspective to learn what stressors are involved. We also need to listen carefully, and to clarify what is being said to determine whether these precipitating, amplifying factors are stressors or distressors. This is an important dimension for you to consider as you sort out your client's modeled world. There are many exciting, stimulating things that happen every day that are stressors. If your client sees them as exciting and positive, that is, perceives them as challenges, it is less likely that the client will identify them as the cause of a health problem. Instead, the client might identify such stressors as a remedy for the problem. On the other hand, stimuli that are seen as distressful are most often associated with interruptions in the health processes. Simply stated, stressors are usually seen as a challenge and distressors are seen as a threat. Both take energy and both can aggregate and culminate in problems for your client. Distressors, however, are more likely to take more energy and cause problems faster than are stressors.

Expectations

The second category for data collection is the expected outcome of the client's situation, that is, what is going to happen. It is useful to consider both what your client thinks will happen immediately and what he or she thinks will happen in the future. Several times we have heard nurses say that some patients simply won't accept what has happened or what lies ahead; they deny that they have a health problem. We note frequently that these people *fear* what they think lies ahead, or what is in their immediate future. Thus, they seem to deny because it seems to them too terrible to think or talk about. Let's take, for example, the case of a woman who was referred to one of us because she was having a great deal of difficulty adjusting to a recent mastectomy. It was suggested that after the nurse completed her consultation with this client, the nurse might enjoy talking to the woman across the hall who also had had a mastectomy. The nurse was informed that the second woman had undergone surgery the same day as the first, but was adjusting exceedingly well. Therefore, it would be "fun" to talk with her.

> Upon entering the first woman's room, the nurse was struck by the anger in the woman's voice as she talked with her husband and daughter. She was somewhat rude to the student nurse in her room and she was, in general, throwing a fit. She was in a hospital gown and looked like someone who had just undergone surgery within the last 48 hours. Her intravenous line was gone, however. After they had talked a few minutes, the nurse determined that the woman was going through a normal grieving process. (After all, who wouldn't be angry?) Her husband and daughter completely understood, and both supported her extremely well. When asked what she thought would happen to her, she said that she would most likely recover "just fine" and be back at work within a month or so. She planned, however, to give herself time to get used to the idea.
>
> The second woman's story was altogether different. She had on a lovely pink negligee, had just plucked her eyebrows,

and was preparing to paint her nails. She was alone and still had an intravenous infusion. When encouraged to express her perceptions, she stated that she didn't think her husband would ever love her again. After all, he had already had other girls on the side, and "who could possibly love a woman with one breast?" She didn't really know if she could handle the future. She couldn't project herself in a loving relationship with anyone, and she could not see herself as worthwhile in any role. The nurse determined that she was wearing makeup and a pretty gown in order to camouflage her feelings. Her medical record showed that this woman required more pain medication than the first (4). Nevertheless, she had been considered to be doing better, just because she "put on a front."

We can be fooled if we don't look and listen holistically. Perhaps, had the nurses talked with this second woman before surgery and asked her what she thought her life would be like in the future, she might have been able to express her awful fear that she would not be worth loving if she really had cancer and had to have a mastectomy. This woman was "denying" the present (if we dare call it denial) only because the present leads to the future. Not many of us would care to see such a gloomy future as she projected for herself, one in which we are not important for anything or to anyone.

A person's expectations of the outcomes of today's stressors are of great importance. How we handle our ongoing stressors is determined partially by what we think will happen as a result of our action and partly by what we think will happen if we do nothing. (We use the word "think" rather loosely here. What we mean is that in most cases people feel or perceive that something will or won't happen, but often they don't really cognitively process the information.)

Research data show that people who are depressed have decreased immune responses (5). We also know that those who are in chronic stress break down protein instead of building it up (6). Because of the implications for healing derived from these facts, we must learn to take into account these mind–body relationships if we are to practice holistic nursing.

Whether or not someone can project himself or herself into the future might be far more important than we know even now. For example, there is the story of a 19-year-old boy, struck with polio in the days before iron lungs, who overheard the doctor tell his mother that he couldn't possibly live until morning. Determined to live, he communicated with his mother, signaling in ways that only she understood, that he wanted his bed and dresser moved so that he could see the sun rise in the mirror. He not only survived that bout with polio but also survived another bout of polio some 20 years later. The two attacks left him breathing with accessory muscles for almost 45 years. Nevertheless, this remarkable man was able to continue to project himself into each tomorrow, to expect that he could control his world, until he succumbed to an overwhelming streptococcal infection at the age of 78. In the interim, though severely crippled and often very ill, he nevertheless continued to grow and develop. At the time of his death, this man was acknowledged as one of the great scholars and teachers of his time (7).

Resource Potential

The third major category of data is that of resource potential. You will need to ask your client where he or she gets support. With whom does the client talk things over? How does the client "keep going"? You will want some information on *potential* resources. Is there anyone who provides reinforcement, helps the client solve problems, and so forth? Does the client have family members or friends nearby and available? Questions like these will indicate your client's social network. It is then necessary to elicit how the client perceives these individuals. The latter point is most important in terms of assessing *support systems*, since there are many families who at first sight seem very reinforcing, but when the client's perspective is asked are revealed to be energy draining rather than energizing. That is, the client perceives that he or she has to do all of the supporting; the client has never really had his or her own dependency needs met very well. Naturally, most people prefer this state of affairs to one in which there is no social network (because people have an innate need for some form of human relationship). Frequently, however, these family members or friends are not providing the kind of support your client wants and needs. Do not misunderstand this point. We are not saying that your client does not want to see these people (although that does happen). Instead, we are saying that you, the nurse, need to know how the client perceives the relationship. Sometimes the client will deplete energy stores trying to maintain a support system when instead he or she should be acquiring, building, and storing energy by interacting with the support system. An *impoverished* person does not have the energy to invest in maintaining others without further depleting his or her own internal resources.

Nurses have known this intuitively for years. In addition to all the reasons for not including families in the care of intensely ill postoperative patients is the knowledge collected by experience that it "wears the patient out." Nurses have seen many patients who have tried to allay the anxieties of their loved ones when the patients should have been receiving the interventions. There are others, however, who perceive their families as vital to their well-being. For example:

> A 28-year-old male who, when confronted with open heart surgery to repair a septal defect and mitral valve insufficiency, requested that his wife (a nurse) have special visiting privileges after surgery. When the request was denied by the health care system, this man went off to surgery with great bravado. He had seemingly accepted his state of affairs. Imagine everyone's surprise when he returned from surgery and refused to speak or understand his own language, but spoke Spanish instead, a language he and his wife had studied together. Since none of the nurses or doctors could understand him, and *he refused to understand them*, his wife was allowed to spend the first 24 hours with him. This was substantially different from the typical five minutes per hour that the health care team had planned for him.

This individual knew what he needed to get well, and he very wisely took control and saw to it that he got what he needed. As a result, he was back on his vigorous job, one that required activity and long hours, less than one month after surgery. Thus, social networks can be considered within the framework of both positive (support) and negative (draining) valences. This is not to say that they are good or bad, but rather to identify their potential for assisting your client in meeting health care needs.

This distinction between a social network, a set of individuals with whom your client is involved, and a support system, a person or persons who provide resources and energize your client, also applies to thinking about your client's relationship with health care providers. You will want to elicit your client's perspective on his or her health care providers, including yourself. The old standby question, "How can I help you help yourself?" is one that we all ask as we try to determine what the client needs from us. Taking the client's response seriously and acting upon it enhances the probability that we will increase our client's resources and available energy rather than further drain or deplete energy stores. You will also want to consider how your client perceives the other members of the health care system so that, again, you can plan interventions that will help the client the most. People who perceive that their doctor or nurse will punish them if they have been "bad" often withhold information that is important in revising medical treatment plans (8). There was, for example, the 17-year-old girl who had been treated in an outpatient health care facility for diabetic control. When her nurse, who had contracted to help her with health care needs—not take care of her diabetes—arrived a few minutes late one day, the girl jumped up with panic on her face and said, "I have to talk to you now." The doctor and clinic nurse were perplexed when she insisted that they leave. As soon as the door was closed, she said, "They were going to increase my insulin. I don't want it to go up. I already have insulin reactions all the time. But my sugar is high this morning, and do you know why? I ate 17 Snickers bars yesterday afternoon. I was having a fight with my mother and just lost my head. Now I'm really going to get it. If I tell the doctor, he'll be really mad, and so will the other nurse. *What can I do?"*

It has been our experience that clients often find themselves in this kind of a bind. They don't know what to do. They're afraid they will be scolded, and so they simply fake the story—and sometimes even leave the health care system. We have learned that very few people stick to the regimens prescribed for them, but far be it from them to tell a doctor or nurse who will scold them for not complying with the medical care plan, a plan that was developed for a disease, not for a person. Most clients would rather have their "order" changed, get "poked" again, and so on, than be found out. It's only after they are certain that we care about them, *not their disease*, that they tell us "the inside story."

Another way to think about this issue is to determine whether your client sees the health care team members as nurturing or controlling. Very few clients are going to openly resist "orders" written by a controlling doctor (or nurse), but not very many are going to follow them explicitly. This is particularly true if the orders are incongruent with the individual's own philosophy in life. Although this point is very important to the total care of a holistic person, we do not want to overemphasize it. We recommend that if you are curious about the health belief model that you read the works of Becker and Rosenstock (9). The point we wish to make is that you want to give some thought to how your client perceives his or her health care resources in order to plan care that will facilitate the client's holistic growth.

In the preceding paragraphs we have discussed the external resources available to the client. We will now turn our attention to those resources that are internal. These strengths fall into two groups: (1) self-strengths and (2) the potential to mobilize resources at a given point in time. Thus strengths might be thought of as being both trait and state in nature. One's ability to mobilize resources for coping with stressors at any given point in time is a state, not a trait. Let's look first at self-strengths which are traits.

When we talk about *self-strengths*, we are referring to all the internal resources that an individual can use to promote health and growth. These strengths can be defined in terms of attitudes, endurance, patterns, or whatever other way you (or your client) choose to define them. Individuals who get great pleasure from music might see their strength in their talent to play, to listen to, to know good music. Others see strength in their appearance, their behaviors toward others, or their ability. If you consider Erikson's developmental stages, with their resulting strengths and virtues, you will get some idea about where these particular characteristics emerge on the normal life span growth grid. What is important is whether or not your client can identify his or her own strengths. Many of our clients are great at listing their weaknesses or limitations but initially have trouble identifying their strengths. Although we could talk about this concept as a part of the person's model, it is too important to bury within another concept. Nurses often find themselves intuitively helping their clients identify what is good or effective about them, what they can buld on, what will help them cope with reality. We urge nurses to continue to do this, but to do so systematically, within the context of a theory base.

Another way to think about internal resources is within the framework of one's current ability to mobilize resources for coping with stressors. This is necessary because stressors create stress. People cannot tolerate prolonged stress states without using up (or severely depleting) their internal energies (10). The resources we are talking about now are both physiological and psychosocial, not just self-strengths as traits. Breathing, for example, is a strength in the case of someone who is fighting for life.

An understanding of an individual's current ability to mobilize coping resources facilitates the nurse's planning of health care. Once the nurse has determined the individual's potential for mobilizing resources and has a sense of how that person models his or her world, the nurse will have a good understanding of the client's ability to mobilize resources to contend with current stressors and the potential effect of future stressors. There are many tragic cases that come to mind wherein an individual's energy could have been saved, and so furthered his or her life, or made that life better, had we considered this concept. Currently, many nurses plan care that is goal-directed, but usually they do so with the objective of immediate problem solving and without consideration for the relationship among the subsystems within the holistic person. It is as though each subsystem were being dealt with in isolation from the other subsystems of the person. This approach does not take into account the interactions among mind, emotion, spirit, and body, or the human potential to shift energy among the various subsystems. Because of this, problems identified within a particular subsystem are often resolved at the cost of creating another problem within the same or another subsystem of the individual.

Drawing energies from one subsystem instead of another does not decrease the energy being used, and it does not arrest the depletion of resources. It simply shifts the burden from one subsystem to another. Overall, holistic persons are still depleting their energy stores. Nursing prescriptions are more purposeful and health-directed when they are made with an understanding of these complex, multisystem interactions and thus with an idea of the individual's ability to mobilize resources at the time. Major intervention differences lie in the handling of people in *arousal* and people in *impoverishment*. Individuals who are *impoverished* require a direct type of care; those who are in *arousal* usually require an indirect approach. The direct type is aimed at meeting affiliation needs, and the indirect approaches are usually aimed at individuation needs. This principle may have exceptions, but it holds true in most cases. These ideas will be expanded in Chapter 11.

Goals and Life Tasks

The final category for consideration as you collect data is that of the goals the individual claims for himself or herself, both immediately and in the future. Some people are too *impoverished* to project themselves very far into the future, and thus sometimes have difficulty with this task. They will say such things as, "All I can think about is taking my next breath." You will know then that their immediate goal is to partially satisfy a physiological need to breathe. Such information is important to the nurse planning care. She needs to know that these individuals are truly at risk, that they will have difficulty mobilizing coping resources. New stressors (or distressors) can be overwhelming. These are the people who develop postoperative infections one after another, and sometimes give up and die.

Generally, however, even those who have trouble projecting an image of themselves into the future can tell you what goals they are struggling with at the time. Sometimes what they want and what they think they should want are two different things. This incongruence, caused by people in the social network urging them to work on one goal while they desire to work on another, generally creates extensive conflict for these individuals and thus increases their distress state.

Nurses need to know what people see as their current and future goals for four main reasons. The first reason is to collect data on an individual's goals in order to identify need deficits. Listening to an individual who states that she can't project herself into the next day and that her only goal is to breathe easier helps the nurse identify basic-need deficits. Ultimately, this will help in planning nursing interventions aimed at these deficits.

The second reason to identify current and future goals is to determine where the client is in the developmental process. As stated earlier, you cannot assume that just because an individual is 45 years of age that person is working on the goals or tasks typically identified for that person's chronological age. Very often this is not the case. Thus, to provide sound nursing interventions, you will need to know what task the client might now need some assistance in working through. Furthermore, identifying life goals helps you determine the level of cognitive processing that you might consider in working with people. Although it may seem strange, there are highly educated people still dealing with their problems within the cognitive framework of a much earlier age. If repeated unmet needs occurred at the stage of autonomy, the associated thinking that occurred at that time characterizes the individual's predominant mode of thinking. Even though the client may now be 50 years old, and may have attained a Ph.D., these experiences did occur together. Knowing this helps the nurse be flexible and creative as she plans interventions for such a client. One client we recall was a middle-aged man who was well advanced, was well known for his work, and was experiencing intractable hypertension. Nursing interventions helped this person achieve a normotensive state.

After listening to his comments and considering his current tasks in life and what he wanted to achieve—as opposed to what his family thought a respectable man of his age and status should achieve—the nurse determined that he had difficulty with affiliated-individuation and was working on the stage of autonomy. During this age in life, people enter into a thinking process that includes animism (that is, they grant life to all things), and they enjoy fantasy. They can also be frightened by their fantasies. They are unable to actually conceptualize, to think logically. Knowing this helped the nurse understand that the client was proceeding through a sequence of concerns about his body (also natural for the two to three-year-old child). He would tell how he felt scared and tense all week and would only feel safe during his time with his nurse. Two things seemed necessary: first, that he would not "accidentally" hurt himself (for example, work himself into a distress state so that a heart attack was imminent); second, he needed something to take with him between sessions that would make him feel safe. Otherwise, he might "have to get sick" in order to have his security, belonging, and esteem needs met.

A contract was written in which he stated that he was not to hurt himself in any way, including having a heart attack (11). In return, he could have an extra period of time with his nurse. (The reward was his choice.) When he left the office, he was handed the contract and carefully told that it was very important and was to serve as a care giver for him until he returned the following week. He was told that this contract had the power to keep him safe and would help him get better soon. The following week he described a very frightening dream (also common for young children ages two to three). He told the nurse that he dared not let his blood pressure get too normal or he wouldn't be able to see her. He was reassured that *she really didn't care about his blood pressure unless he was concerned about it* and that *she was interested only in him.* He commented that he'd better carry his contract with him another week or so. The following week he was normotensive. Approximately one year later, this client told his nurse that he still had his contract, and that, although he knew there was no longer a danger of his hurting himself, he still liked to have that "silly piece of paper that saved my life."

This man, very bright and well educated, benefited from the nurse's knowledge that animism is normal for small children. Such magical thinking had worked against him at another time, but now it was put to work for him.

The third reason to collect data on your client's perceptions about goals and life tasks is so that you will be better able to plan interventions that are within *the client's* model, not someone else's. There are many children who have taken piano lessons, swimming lessons, and so forth, because their mothers wanted them to acquire such skills. Sometimes forcing our goals on our client is not useful and sometimes it creates an additional stressful event.

The final reason to listen to your client's plans for the future is that it will provide you with information to predict where your client is headed. If you aggregate your information in terms of basic needs, developmental tasks, and object relations, you will be able to determine whether or not growth can be predicted.

THE NURSE'S OBSERVATIONS

We need to talk about the nurse's observations here, although we have commented about our observations throughout the book. We hope you will bear with us.

The nurse makes continuous observations as she works with her client. She collects verbal and nonverbal data, frequently checking with her client concerning his or her perspective on these observations. Sometimes, however, she chooses to store the data and discuss it with the client at a later time. At other times she makes observations that she does not ever check with her client directly. For example, a very *impoverished* person may fear new knowledge. The nurse may note that this is possible. To ask the client directly if her perception is accurate might only result in increased impoverishment. In this case, it would be more useful for the nurse to tell the individual that she can provide information about the topic to be taught, and that if and when the client would like that information she would be happy to share it. She might also say that she knows that some people are sometimes frightened or concerned about receiving such information and others are not. She might add that this is normal, and that it is best for each person to decide what he or she wants to know and when he or she wants to know it. Furthermore, there are some things that those who are frightened might do to help themselves, such as holding someone's hand, having a special person with them, holding a pillow or good luck charm, *whatever would make them feel safest.* The nurse would probably want to reemphasize that the person knows what's best for himself or herself, and that the nurse is eager to help the person do what is best.

You will probably want to categorize your observations, just as you have those of your client and the client's support system. This will help you to be systematic and thorough. For that reason, we will make a few comments about each category listed.

Description of the Situation

You will make observations of the situation and formulate causative relationships. In some instances, you will find that your observations clearly indicate those causative relationships; in others, you will want to collect more data before you make a diagnosis. You can continue to collect data as you continue your interactive, interpersonal nursing process. In addition to these factors related to your immediate observation, you might also want to consider other possibilities, since you will be able to predict what could happen if you use your knowledge of the mind–body relationship. For example, people run out of energy and need to be restored; basic needs are innate; and so on. You may also want to speculate on some nursing interventions that might be useful given these relationships.

One thing you will want to keep in mind is that you are making nursing observations, not medical observations. Although both nurse and doctor might be interested in the same phenomena, you have different reasons for your interest and thus will note different relationships. For example, you might be working with a client who has recently undergone surgery. The doctor will be interested in the physiological status of the wound: "Is it healing? Is it infected?" The doctor's major concern is that the wound is not infected, that it doesn't have "something wrong with it." You, too, are interested in the wound because it is a part of the person with whom you are working. You are interested in all of the "right" things about the wound. How healthy and strong does the tissue seem to be? How well is it healing? More importantly, though, you are concerned with how your client feels and thinks about that wound. What does it represent to the client? What does the client expect will happen as a result of the surgery? And so on. Your observations will be made in terms of the holistic person, and they will be based on your knowledge of normal human beings' biophysical systems, basic needs, and developmental stages. The doctor's observations and diagnoses will be made in terms of illness, disease, and abnormality.

Expectations

Your observations about your client's expectations are important. While clients sometimes say that they expect one thing, their body language may suggest something else. You will want to keep this in mind as you continue to observe your client over time. Perhaps an incongruence exists with families, role expectations, and so on, that undermines the individual's own expectations, no matter how positive they might be initially. You will also want to take into account your expectations of the situation.

We have known cases in which the nurse seemed to give up on the individual, which seemed to result in the client's giving up. There have also been cases in which nurses continued to provide holistic, health-producing care, in spite of client and medical staff expectations, and the people got well (12).

Resource Potential

You will make observations about your client's external and internal resources. Since the nurse does things with, for, and on the behalf of her client, these observations will help her to think about her client's total needs. Does the client seem to have a positive, supportive family, or not? That is, do they seem to restore the energy level of your client, or does the client seem depleted after these visits? How do the doctor and the client interact? How does the client interact with other health care members? Does your client seem to need some help in working with these individuals? These are all the observations that you might make, and check out, with your client.

You will observe your client's physical status and feeling state. You will note when the client makes repeated comments about being tired, sluggish, burned out, sad, depressed, slow, anxious, and so forth. You will want such information because you are determining what resources your client has available for coping.

Goals and Life Tasks

Your goals for your client should be clear in your mind. When you keep developmental stages and tasks, strengths, and virtues associated with each stage in mind, you will have a sense of the direction in which you want your client to progress. Naturally, since you must first determine where the client is presently, you will want to observe the goals he or she seems to be working toward and the tasks the client is working on. Once you know these, you can predict what tasks will likely emerge next. We have heard nurses (particularly those who work with clients over long periods of time) say, "Just as you get one problem taken care of, another comes up." We think this statement reflects a lack of understanding that resolution of one developmental task *automatically* means that new tasks will emerge. That's human nature.

This doesn't mean that your client is having one *problem* after another; instead, the client is working through one *task* after another. True, the client may try to work on these tasks in the same maladaptive manner that characterized his or her first attempt at working through this stage, and therefore seems to be having a problem. If you can keep this state of affairs in mind, your goals will be directed toward *positive task resolution*, and there will be decreased conflict about its resolution. We have observed middle-aged individuals begin with the stage of autonomy and work through the various stages to the appropriate tasks for their age. Take, for example, the same individual mentioned earlier who, at the age of 50, began to work on the developmental task of autonomy and then proceeded through each stage until he reached the stage of generativity. At each new encounter, he would return to his nurse to reassure himself that his goals in life were appropriate and acceptable. We recall that one day he came in, tense and concerned. Finally, he talked about his (current) problem. He had just realized that while he still treasured his intimate relationship with his wife, he was more interested in writing his book, reporting his life's work, than he was in this relationship. Our response was "Hallelujah!" You're now entering the stage of generativity." Clearly, if this man's intimate relationship with his wife had been threatened, he would not have felt the freedom to move forward.

Nurses who are concerned with life-span development will want to keep the goals and tasks of the various stages in mind as they interpret data. This will help them predict where their clients will move next and they will be able to help their clients anticipate potential trouble when they seem to be moving backward instead of forward.

THE FAMILY AND FRIENDS' OBSERVATIONS

When you collect data from family members and friends, you will want to follow the same general format you did when you collected data from the client. That is, you will want to collect information in the four categories as described in the model. Remember, your goal is to collect data from the family's perspective, not to invalidate or validate your client's perspective. Naturally, you will consider the congruence between the two sources when you analyze the data. Furthermore, you will note specific factors that your client's family focuses on while providing the data. These have to do with the concept of affiliated-individuation. Specifically, you will be interested in the family's thoughts on how the client's situation impacts on him or her and how it changes family roles and plans.

Description of the Situation

You will want to know what factors are involved in the client's current situation from the family's perspective. You will be interested in whether the family perceives these factors as stressors or distressors, as challenging or threatening, and how they interrelate with other family member's lives and needs. When you collect data on therapeutic interventions you will be interested in what family members think will make the client healthier and in how that will impact other family members. Many times families do not give members permission to have their needs met because it is perceived that it will have a greater negative effect on other family members or the family as a whole. If this is the case, you will need to know about it before you can plan holistic care. In most cases, an individual's desire for affiliated-individuation is associated with the family. We have known several individuals who, in meeting their own needs, seemed to deprive other family members of their need satisfaction. When this happened, our clients often withdrew from personal need satisfaction goals in order to meet those family members' needs. This means that there are families in which one member assumes the role of care taker while others accept the role of care receivers (13).

When the care taker encounters a situation in which he or she must switch roles, there is often difficulty within the *family as a system.* A major problem is that there is no other care giver in such a family. The care taker "takes care of" the family, controlling, planning, and doing for family members. Other family members function only as care receivers and expect care to be given to them. These families lack someone to nurture, accept, and give care that will help the individual members of the family gain autonomy, while still giving permission to have dependency needs met. They do not understand the principle embedded in the statement "If you love something, let it go, for if it was really love it will return. If it does not, it was not love to start." For they are fearful that their care taker will not return. These families require expert nursing care that will provide nurturance directed at various members of the family: that is, role-modeling that shows members that it is possible for all members to meet both affiliation and individuation needs.

In short, what we are talking about overlaps with the resources category of data collection. You will discover that the family's perception of what is supportive to your client might be an important key to the distressors in the situation. We have known families whose members have stated that the client attained support from keeping his or her job. There is certainly something to be said about esteem and security needs being met through one's job, but it is also possible that the job is especially important because love and belonging needs are not adequately satisfied. This situation is aggravated by the fact that many such individuals will state that their problems are caused by stress on the job. You will be able to understand these relationships and your client better as you keep in mind the concepts set forth in Chapters 4 and 5.

Expectations

Remembering that your client wants affiliated-individuation and usually wants the family to provide the primary source of support, you will need to know what the family expects will happen, both to your client and to them. These data are important, for if you remember Maslow's words about knowledge—there is both the need to know and the fear of knowing—you will know that many families are so fearful of knowing the truth, and at the same time desperately need to know, that they develop a set of "truths" for themselves, or simply pretend that nothing is happening. In either case, if your client wants to talk to the family about the situation, he or she may become locked into a pattern of dysfunctional communications. Such a situation isolates your client (14) and results in unmet basic needs. Sometimes the basic-need deficits are so great that the individual becomes physically ill (15). (You might review the section on the mind–body continuum if this statement doesn't make sense to you. Remember, people have a hierarchy of needs. When the psychosocial needs are unmet, energies are drawn from the physical subsystem and can tax it to the point of sickness.)

Resource Potential

We have already started a discussion on resource potential, but now we will elaborate a bit more. Family members will provide some insights into both internal and external resources as you collect data about your client. They can give their perceptions on your client's usual coping mechanisms, how the client views the health care team, when the client is willing to seek assistance, what the client's strengths are, how the client seems to have been feeling lately. Sometimes these points are very important, for frequently individuals do not recognize that their social networks attend to such issues. We have had several clients who were amazed to hear the family members' perspectives on their strengths. In some cases, strengths were identified by the client as weaknesses. Such perceptions can help change a "wormy looking creature into a caterpillar about to become a beautiful butterfly." Support systems sometimes notice when people are not their usual selves even before the individuals do. When this happens, you as the nurse can use the data to help your client try to determine what might have been going on that the family noticed that he or she didn't; that is, what was happening that may have been stressful or distressful. Such information helps both you and your client plan wisely for the future.

Goals and Life Tasks

You will want to learn what the family perceives your client's goals to be, both for now and for the future. As mentioned earlier, there are many situations in which a person is working on an earlier life task while the family thinks he or she should be working on something else. Take, for example, the man whose family states that he gets his support from the job and never seems to need or interact with the family. He seems only interested in making money. This individual may have been working on the stages of initiative and industry at the cost of working on the stage of intimacy and generativity. Sometimes this information can provide important clues for the nurse who keeps in mind that her client *wants to be the best that he or she can be and wants affiliated-individuation.*

In general, we can say that families are important sources of data because they will provide insights into our clients that we might not otherwise obtain. These data will help us to speculate about incongruencies in relationships and communication patterns. These incongruencies create distress for our clients, deplete their energy, and often result in maladaptive coping patterns.

THE MEDICAL TEAM'S OBSERVATIONS

There will be times when you will want to incorporate the medical team's observations and plans in your data bank. Such information will help you provide information to your client and will also help you better understand your client's perspective. You will probably discover that you can collect medical information about the description of the situation, and (perhaps) the expectations. We hasten to point out that this is true not because of neglect or lack of caring, but simply because these health practitioners focus on the disease, sickness, and conditions, instead of on the holistic person. Thus, most physicians collect and interpret data from the perspective of sickness, disease, or injury. We believe that this is appropriate and that as colleagues we should be willing to assist them in achieving their goals, just as we expect them to assist us in achieving our goals of promoting holistic health (16).

OTHERS' OBSERVATIONS

Nurses interested in holistic care will include data from all health care providers who seem to impact on the care of the individual. We will not elaborate on each section of data here, but we do encourage you to keep in mind the potential for incongruence among the various data bases. The nurse is the *only* health care provider who is responsible for holistic care. As such, she naturally takes all perspectives into account in order to be certain that interventions, goals, and expectations are congruent with those of the client.

Our focus is to make the total environment as conducive as possible to meeting the client's needs and promoting the client's welfare. We are not interested in helping other health care team members meet their goals just for the sake of helping them. Our aim is to help them so that they can help our client, if and when our client so desires.

COLLECTING THE DATA

The first part of this chapter discussed what you should think about as you collect data. This section provides a few pointers on how to collect data. We do not perceive this discussion as inclusive, but we do hope it will stimulate your thoughts. It is our view that the data-collection phase of the nursing process starts with the person, giving your utmost attention to the person's perspective. By this we mean that you start with the person's stated concerns and stay with these concerns until the person changes the focus of the interaction. Data collection is usually confined to the details needed to get the client's full perception of his or her concern and to the data (physical and otherwise) needed to understand the situation so that plans can be made that will facilitate a movement toward the comfort, healing, or health goal.

At the beginning of every client or patient contact, we invite clients to share with us their worries, questions, or concerns. We engage active listening skills, taking seriously both verbal and nonverbal messages without being judgmental. We *never discount* what a person says, especially not in favor of any personal interpretation of the meaning of nonverbal messages. If we choose to work directly with nonverbal messages (by necessity if a client is unable to speak), we describe the nonverbal behavior and ask the client what it means. The client must validate any possible interpretations we make of those meanings. We accept both verbal and nonverbal messages as equally valid and important, each reflecting various aspects of the person's *unique model* of his or her world or experience. In other words, we do not believe that nonverbal language is necessarily more honest or accurate.

The story comes to mind of the psychiatrist who was watching a child playing outside. When the psychiatrist saw the child break an angleworm into two parts, he assumed that this was an aggressive and sadistic act. He then confronted the child and asked him why he had done such a thing. He was enlightened when the child, in all innocence, said that he felt sorry for the worm having no one to play with and had made him a playmate by creating the second worm! (17).

We take verbal comments at face value and we also ask ourselves while we listen to the client, "What is the client saying?" "What is the client feeling?" Our intention is to identify the client's full perception of the topic under discussion. To do this, we elicit as completely as possible the connotative meanings the client assigns to the things and events being discussed. We also try to garner the feelings the client is experiencing. We avoid imposing upon the client our own model of people and events which might distort our understanding of the client's world because such distortions interfere with establishing an effective, interactive, and interpersonal relationship.

We remember that a problem well defined is a problem half solved. We define problems through standard communication skills: reflecting, clarifying, focusing, summarizing, requesting examples and details. We use the traditional "What if ... ?" "What prevents you from ... ?" "What would happen if ... ?" "What's the worst thing that could happen?" "What control do you have over that worst thing?" We place heavy emphasis on questions that begin with how, what, and in what way. Questions like these help clients change nouns into verbs and to attach feelings to associated events. This, in turn, helps clients realize that effects, behaviors, thoughts, and situations they may have considered unyielding may indeed be changeable or negotiable. We try to catch both conscious and unconscious assumptions, and then ask for validation with such comments as, "It seems that there might be some concern about...." We try never to say, "You are concerned with..." or "You just said that...." Such statements are often seen as too confronting and nonaccepting of the individual's world. Although we may be right, the client might not personally like that characteristic about himself or herself and would therefore assume that we wouldn't like it.

Whatever answer is given to these inquiries is important, and it should be accepted. It is a part of the client's model of the world. The comment or response "I don't know," usually means that the person isn't ready to pursue a given thought or topic.

We try to be affirming and reinforcing whenever our clients show self-disclosure and positive growth. We also attempt to affirm and reinforce every client in some way during our discussions. For example, at the very least, we can genuinely say that we like the way a person "doesn't seem to have all the answers" or "is aware that she wants something (even though she isn't sure yet what it is)." We know that such statements, while affirming, can also be considered embedded commands (18). That is, the client will hear the comment and tuck it away in the mind, later to unconsciously begin working toward health and growth. The comment "You don't act like you know all the answers" carries the unspoken counterpart, "You do have some of the answers."

We often mirror the client's body language, vocal tones, pace and inflections to speed up or slow down a conversation and to better establish rapport. When the person is in conflict, we hope to lead him or her gradually toward a wider, redefined, "reframed," more constructive, or more comfortable restructuring of his or her current perceptions. We use metaphors and analogies freely, such as "the cup may be seen as half-full or half-empty." We also know that variation in our choice of words, tones, facial expressions, and movements is acceptable. This is because we are trying to model our client's world, instead of using a standard format for communication.

At all times we promote and seek to use communication that is open, warm, honest, direct, and kind. In the final analysis, this may be the single most important key to personal survival, growth, and optimal health for clients and care givers alike! It is certainly the only means by which a full-orbed interpersonal trusting relationship can develop as we offer people our professional assistance. When the thoughts, feelings, and behaviors of both care giver and care receiver are handled by the nurse with the deepest respect, the stage is set for negotiations that will bring maximum benefit to each party in the transaction.

Our approach of starting where the person is—by inviting the person to express his or her own most pressing questions, worries, or concerns—deserves special emphasis. Unless the client is totally unaware of or not attending to a life-threatening phenomenon, *his or her own personal concern takes top priority* for our nursing attentions. This does not mean that we ignore simultaneous concerns, of which we only may be aware. It does mean that we respect our client's own timing and patiently await an expression of his or her wanting to deal with a particular observation, action, or learning, unless, of course, a delay or omission of attention places the person in *known and certain* jeopardy. If an unattended medical need or some ill-considered course needs to be brought to the client's, doctor's, or someone else's immediate attention, we feel free to express that concern as *our* concern. We take responsibility for sharing with the client our knowledge of the sciences and clinical judgment of the situation as it is currently. Our constant thrust here is that nursing care should be given as an interactive, interpersonal process in which the client perceives himself or herself as a deeply respected participant-executor to the greatest possible extent in the decisions affecting his or her care.

These paragraphs were presented in order to present a guide for data collection and stimulate your thinking about the use of communication skills and theory in nursing. We feel that these are some of the most important skills a nurse can have, though they are often shortchanged since we have not yet learned how important it is to listen wisely. We do not propose to offer a complete model for communication in these few pages. Rather, we hope to offer some food for thought and some enticement for continued development of communication skills. If you are interested in seeking more information about communication theory and skills, we refer you to the chapter bibliography at the back of the book.

SUMMARY

In this chapter we have suggested that there are three sources of data for you to consider. Your primary source is your client; information obtained from the client comes through your having developed an interactive and interpersonal working relationship with the client to assist the client to attain and maintain optimum health, given his or her circumstances. Secondary sources of data include your own nursing observations and information provided by family and friends. Tertiary sources of data include the physician's observations and plans and other health professionals' observations and plans. Often tertiary information is obtained from the client's medical record; in other instances, you might prefer to confer directly with health professionals. Four kinds of data need to be collected from these various sources. You will want information about the description of the situation, expectations, resource potential, and goals and life tasks. Your client, of course, can provide you with information within all four categories. Other sources will not be so comprehensive, but it is important to keep all four categories of data in mind when you turn to secondary and tertiary sources for information. In the next chapter we will discuss what to do with the information you have collected.

1. You may wish to review the concept of *impoverishment* as a state in the adaptive potential assessment model in Chapter 5.

2. These interventions consisted of teaching this man how to imagine that he was conversing with his nurse about his daily stressors and distressors. He was encouraged to consider the possible alternatives that he might have as he continued dealing with these phenomena and to remember that his nurse was "really only a telephone away" at almost all times. These interventions were designed only after the client began to express an interest and desire to be independent of his nurse.

3. Separation-individuation is Mahler's way of describing the process of resolving the task of autonomy. A good reference is C. Schuster and S. Ashburn, *The Process of Human Development: A Holistic Approach* (Boston: Little, Brown and Co., 1980).

4. Follow-up showed that this woman also experienced a slower recovery rate than her neighbor. She was on intravenous feedings longer, ambulated slower, and exercised her arm less than the first woman did.

5. R. W. Bartrop, L. Lazarus, E. Luckhurst, L. G. Kiloh, and R. Penny, "Depressed Lymphocyte Function After Bereavement." *The Lancet* 1 (1977): 834–36.

6. A. Vander, J. Sherman, and D. Luciano, *Human Physiology*, 2d ed. (New York: McGraw-Hill, 1975), pp. 499–502.

7. This story is about Milton H. Erickson and was told by both him and his mother. As stated in Chapter 7, note 1, Dr. Erickson provided provocative insights into modeling and role-modeling. He often stated that every nurse and doctor should be confined to a wheelchair for one month of their education so that they would learn how important it is to understand the *client's world*.

8. For more information on the "good patient phenomenon," see *Patients, Physicians, and Illness: A Source Book in Behavioral Science and Health*, 3d ed. (New York: Free Press, 1979).

9. Marshall Becker, *The Health Belief Model and Personal Health Behavior* (Thorofare, N.J.: Charles B. Slack, 1974). I. Rosenstock, "Why People Use Health Services," *Milbank Memorial Fund Quarterly* 44 (1966): 94–124.

10. You will remember that Selye has shown that the maximum time that the alarm reaction can be maintained in 72 hours. If the

individual does not experience relief from the stressor or receive additional resources, the individual will move to the exhaustive stage within a short time.

11. The underlying assumptions with this intervention are that the individual was working on the stage of autonomy during which persons need to feel safe and certain that they will be taken care of if necessary and that they will not be allowed to "lose control." Just as the care giver would not allow a small child to play with dangerous toys, this nurse would not encourage her client to "act out physiologically" to the extent that he was physically endangered. Thus, she stated, "I need to know that you will be safe for the next week . . . that you won't do anything to harm yourself, including having a heart attack. If you should meet my needs, what would you like in return?"

This intervention implicitly informed this client that he was important, worthwhile, and valued and that he had the potential to take "good" (not bad) care of himself.

12. We have all seen situations in which the nurse or family will not emotionally give up and the client responds. We have seen several such cases, one of which was discussed in Chapter 5 in the section on adaptation potential.

13. A good resource for more information about families is Marilyn Friedman, *Family Nursing* (Englewood Cliffs, N.J.: Prentice-Hall, 1981).

14. Many people experiencing the grief process have described themselves as "alone, isolated, unable to talk with anyone" about their lives and what they expected would happen. Colin Murray Parkes provides important insights into interventions for these individuals in his book *Bereavement: Studies of Grief in Adult Life* (New York: International University Press, Inc., 1972).

15. Colin Parkes reports his and others' findings on this concept in *Bereavement: Studies of Grief in Adult Life*. See note 14.

16. Nurses do have such expectations. We ask the doctor to talk with the patient about the illness problem when our client indicates that he or she wants to talk with the doctor, or we ask the doctor to include the family, and so forth. This is not the doctor's primary concern or role in health care, but as a colleague, he or she is willing to help us achieve our goals just as we help the doctor with his or hers.

17. The original source of this story is lost to the authors. We

heard it from Milton Erickson as an example of how essential modeling is if we are to understand our clients' needs.

18. If you are interested in more information on "embedded commands," we again refer you to the work of Milton Erickson. A subsidiary source is Richard Bandler and John Grinder, *Patterns of the Hypnotic Techniques of Milton H. Erickson*, M.D., volume 1 (Cupertino, California: Meta Publications, 1975), pp. 172–178.

10

How Does One Aggregate, Analyze, and Synthesize Data?

OVERVIEW

We addressed the data-collection phase of the nursing process in Chapter 9 and briefly discussed some communication techniques and concepts. This chapter will consider what to do with the data you collect. Before you can begin to analyze the data, you will need to pull together the information you have gained from your primary, secondary, and tertiary sources for each of the four major categories of data: description of the situation, expectations, resource potential, and goals and life tasks. Once you have compiled the data, you will search for relationships within the data that will lead to interpretations, diagnoses, and the formulation of goals for intervention. This chapter will discuss in detail how to complete this phase of the nursing process.

PERSPECTIVES

There are a few thoughts you will need to keep in mind as you read this chapter. First, you are a nurse, not a doctor. Therefore, you will not need to make medical diagnoses. You will aggregate and analyze data for the sole purpose of making nursing diagnoses. Second, you have most of what you need to know to practice this paradigm. You have from previous readings or experiences, most of the knowledge stored in your conscious and subconscious minds. You are already making nursing diagnoses, such as those described here. Sometimes you communicate your diagnoses to others; sometimes you don't. Sometimes you have *objective* data to support your diagnoses; sometimes you don't. No matter—you have a *practice* paradigm. Perhaps your practice model is very much like our structured, labeled paradigm but it is less structured and it lacks the labels, articulation, and direction. If so, you will have no difficulty in aggregating data. You've been doing it all along. If not, you will become expert with practice. This chapter provides an organizational format and a system that will help you to be more consistent and to describe what you've done.

What, then, do you need to aggregate, analyze, and synthesize data within the modeling and role–modeling paradigm?(1) First, you must learn how to do this from the perspective of holism. We have said that the individual is a total person with a mind–body relationship and that our goal is to nurture our consumer to the maximum possible state of holistic health, growth, and development. Therefore, you cannot think of data from one particular subsystem exclusively. Nor can you think of it from a problem-oriented perspective exclusively. When we aggregate data in terms of subsystems, we most frequently conclude with a diagnosis that considers only one domain (or subsystem) of the individual and does not consider the dynamic holism of the human being. The problem-oriented approach frequently (implicitly and explicitly) excludes the individual's strengths. Instead, the focus is often on deficits, weaknesses, and problems. Finally, neither approach emphasizes *self-care knowledge* as taking precedence over all other knowledge bases.

The second thing that will help you aggregate and analyze data in the modeling and role–modeling paradigm most effectively is to acquire a reasonable understanding of the theoretical formulations presented in Chapters 4 through 6. If you do not have such a knowledge base at this time, don't clutch. We know from experience that you can practice this paradigm by simply following the major principles involved and remembering the aims of interventions (presented in Chapter 11). We have have a case in which this paradigm was used "long distance" by a biologist who was caring for her mother.

The biologist called us and provided the client data we needed, was given the principles and aims, and was encouraged to apply them within the framework of the paradigm. In this manner, she was able to promote holistic nursing care in a hospital about 700 miles from us. As a result, she was able to help her mother regain her health, leave the hospital, and finally move to a new location of her choice.

Undergraduate sophomore students have similar experiences. They certainly are not experts on all of the theories presented herein, but they can easily practice nursing from this paradigm. We do, however, encourage you to continue to seek new insights and gain new knowledge. To do this, you will need to read the works of the authors cited. You will probably gain new perspectives, and new understandings of their work. As a result, you will be able to collect, aggregate, and analyze your data with much greater ease.

If you use our paradigm, you can analyze data and make diagnoses within the framework set forth in the chapter on data collection. To refresh your memory, there are four major categories for data collection: description of the situation, expectations, resource potential, and goals and life tasks. We will follow this same format as we consider the aggregation and analyses of data collected from the biophysical and psychosocial being—your client—the client's family and friends, the nurses, the doctors, and all others involved.

Before beginning data analysis, you will want to aggregate all the data you have collected. Naturally, it is possible that the only sources from which you will have drawn may be your client (and the client's self-care knowledge base) and your own observations. If this is the case, your aggregation process will incorporate these two data sets and nothing more. As you collect more data you will go back and reaggregate, reanalyze, and conclude whether or not your new data warrant a change in plans. This is inherent in the expression *nursing process.* You will constantly keep in mind the holistic framework for nursing. This means that sometimes you will have to make decisions that will seem incongruent with your past socialization. For example, there may be times when you will collect the data and then discover that the client is working from perspectives and toward goals that differ from those of the doctor, the family, or even yourself. When this happens, you must consider your client's holistic nature, the concepts of basic needs, and life-span growth. Then you will determine whether your client is directed toward a healthier, more holistic health state with his or her plan, as compared to the plans of others. If you determine that the client's plan is really best, in spite of the fact that most health care professionals think it isn't, you might be forced either to support your client's self-care knowledge or to revert to practicing under an old "medical model" for nursing in which the client is a patient and the focus is the sickness or condition. Let us give you an example, the case of the biologist and her mother mentioned above.

> The biologist's mother announced most straightforwardly that her state of affairs was a result of her feeling alone and afraid. She stated that she needed a sitter to help her get well, that she would not get well unless she got a sitter, and that she wanted to be dependent and taken care of immediately. Her nurses and doctors (all in a well-known rehabilitation unit in a large hospital) were dismayed. They wanted her to take control of her life, to get up and around, to be independent. They did not want her to have a sitter. They thought she should be getting better by all ordinary expectations but noted that she was deteriorating and didn't know what to do. Her daughter—believing that people who are holistic and growth-oriented can also be *impoverished*—was willing and eager to support her mother's *self-care knowledge* rather than the opinion of the health care providers. (We must state that initially the daughter had agreed with all the others and had spent a great deal of time and money supporting the doctors and nurses in their efforts to meet *their* goals and satisfy their expectations.) As reported earlier, the final outcome was well worth a change in approach by all. The nurses and doctors, convinced that the woman was merely going down hill at a rapid rate were willing to "temporarily" allow a sitter. When this woman was asked how long she thought she would need the sitter, she said that she didn't know. (This response, of course, worried the nurses who feared that she would become "dependent" on a sitter.) However, when asked *when she thought she would be ready to decide how long she would need a sitter*, she readily agreed that she would be ready in two days. Using this approach, the nurses were able to meet her basic needs, provide her with control over her life, establish a trusting relationship, and thus encourage her to move into equilibrium and toward better health.

Nurses are constantly confronted with these difficult decisions. Often we decide in the client's favor, but we can't explain why from a theoretical perspective. As you become more and more aware of the concepts and theoretical formulations we have described, you will be better able to talk with all members of the health care team to state explicitly why you make your decisions. Sometimes your colleagues will disagree with your decision, even though you may have articulated your theory well. Many excellent nurses occasionally find themselves in this position. At such times, the nurse must decide *for* whom she works and *with* whom she works. No matter for whom the nurse works, in our opinion, it is important that she work *with the client*.

Once you have aggregated the data, that is, compiled the data you want to analyze, you will begin to search for relationships among the data (analysis) that will help you make interpretations and diagnoses (synthesis). You will do this by considering all of your data within the four major categories previously described. That is, you

TABLE 10-1   Format for Analysis and Synthesis

Data Categories	Interpretation	Diagnosis
Description of the Situation		
1. Overview of the situation		
2. Etiology		
Stressors		
Distressors		
3. Therapeutic needs		
Expectations		
1. Immediate		
2. Long-term		
Resource Potential		
1. External		
Social network		
Support system		
Health care system		
2. Internal		
Self-strengths		
Adaptive potential		
Feeling states		
Physiological states		
Goals and Life Tasks		
1. Current		
2. Planned		

will want to consider the description of the situation, expectations, potential resources, and goals and life tasks. We explicitly discuss each of these below. You will find key questions to consider in each category.

Table 10-1 shows a format for data analysis and synthesis. Tables 10-2 through 10-5 present detailed information about each category of data and show how it all fits together. Chapter 11 will help you consider nursing interventions that relate to these concepts.

DESCRIPTION OF THE SITUATION

This category has three major focuses for you to consider as you analyze and synthesize the data. You will be concerned with:

1. Developing an overview of the situation
2. Identifying etiological factors involved
3. Identifying possible therapeutic interventions

There are several questions you will ask and many concepts and theoretical bases you will consider as you aggregate and analyze data to achieve the above objectives. These questions and concepts are shown in Table 10-2. You will note that they primarily address the client's perspective, but this does not mean that you will ignore the other sources of data. Instead, it means that you will consider all data but keep the client's *self-care knowledge* foremost in your mind.

As you analyze the data, within the context of the relevant concepts and theoretical bases identified, you will make both interpretations and diagnoses with intervention goals in mind. Thus, you have an interpretive purpose that interfaces with your intervention goal. Stated another way, you will have a reason for analyzing your data using specific conceptual and theoretical bases. Ultimately, these interpretations affect your ability to plan interventions that have a predictable outcome.

Your goal for interpretive purposes will be to describe the situation, its cause and possible therapeutic interventions, keeping in mind all sources of data. Your diagnoses will specify the etiological factors involved in the situation, the need for information, and possible therapeutic interventions.

TABLE 10-2 Description of the Situation

Data Category Focuses	Aggregation and Analysis	
	Questions	Concepts and Theoretical Bases
1. Overview of the situation	1.1 What is the client's perception of the situation?	Self-care: personal model
	1.2 Is it congruent with the perception of the other sources of information?	
	1.3 What is the mind–body relationship?	Dynamic holism
	Which subsystems are involved?	Adaptation
	1.4 Are there basic-need deficits?	Lifetime growth: basic needs
	1.5 Are there growth-need deficits?	
2. Etiological factors	2.1 What etiological factors are involved? Are they stressors? Distressors? Are they threatening or challenging?	Adaptation potential: stress versus distress
	2.2 What factors are associated with the stressors and distressors?	Inherent endowment
	2.3 Are there any losses associated?	Affiliated-Individuation
	2.4 Are the losses real, threatened, or perceived?	
	2.5 Are the losses recent or distant?	
3. Therapeutic needs	3.1 What will help this person get well or healthier?	Self-care: personal model
	3.2 What are the possible objects that could be utilized to satisfy basic-need deficits?	Dynamic holism Adaptation Affiliated-Individuation
	3.3 Is there a need to know or fear of knowing?	Lifetime growth: basic needs

	Synthesis	
Interpretive Purpose	Diagnoses	Long-Term Intervention Goal
1. Development of a *client model* of the situation, including an overview perspective of the client's situation	*Description* of the functional relationship among the factors (2)	Developing a trusting, functional relationship between yourself and your client
2. Etiological factors involved	*Stressors* and *distressors* Stress state	
3. Possible therapeutic interventions as well as possible conflict with treatment plan of other professionals	Possible therapeutic interventions Status of need for information	

Your long-term intervention goal will be to develop a trusting, interactive, and interpersonal nursing relationship between yourself and your client. Table 10-2 shows the relationships among the interpretive purpose, the diagnoses, and the intervention goal within the category of description of the situation.

EXPECTATIONS

This category has three major focuses for you to consider as you aggregate and analyze data:

1. Identifying your client's expectations for the immediate future
2. Identifying your client's expectations for the long-range future
3. Determining the congruency of these expectations (that is, numbers 1 and 2 above) with those of other data sources

Your primary concern is whether or not your client can project himself or herself into the future, and specifically, what the client perceives as the natural outcome of his or her current state. You will be concerned with whether or not the client's projections are health-producing and whether or not they concur with data collected from other sources. The latter point is of particular importance when your client has a negative projection and others do not. Incongruency among the data bases mandates that you intervene *if and when such incongruency interferes with your client's basic-need satisfaction.* Specific questions and relevant concepts and theoretical bases are given in Table 10-3.

Aggregating and analyzing data to determine your client's personal orientation, both immediately and in a long-range time span will be done in order to establish a model of your client's world. Your interpretive purpose will be to determine your client's ability to project himself or herself into the future and to determine the nature of that projection. Your diagnoses will specify your client's personal orientation; your intervention goal will facilitate your client's futuristic and positive self-projections. The relationships among interpretive purpose, diagnoses, and intervention goals for the category expectations are also given in Table 10-3.

TABLE 10-3 Expectations

Data Category Focuses	Aggregation and Analysis			Synthesis		
	Questions	Concepts and Theoretical Bases	Interpretive Purpose	Diagnosis	Long-Term Intervention Goals
1. Immediate expectations	1.1 What does the client think will happen to him or her today? 1.2 What does the client see as the outcome of today's interventions? 1.3 Questions 1.1 and 1.2 for next 48 hours. 1.4 How does the client imagine the nurse–client relationship will evolve? 1.5 Can the client project himself or herself into the future? 1.6 How far into the future? 1.7 What is the image? 1.8 Is the image (projection) growth-directed? 1.9 What are the associated factors?	Self-care: personal model	Development of an understanding of the client's personal orientation in terms of the client's expectations for the future	Personal orientation	Facilitating a self-projection that is futuristic and positive (3)
2. Long-term expectations	2.1 How far can the client project himself or herself? 2.2 What is the long-term expected outcome? 2.3 Can the client project affiliated-individuation? 2.4 Can the client project growth and development? 2.5 What are the associated factors?				

RESOURCE POTENTIAL

This category has two major focuses for you to consider:

1. Identifying your client's external resources
2. Identifying your client's internal resources

As you analyze and aggregate data in order to determine your client's external and internal resource potential, you will be concerned with the client's relationships with the family, friends, and health care providers. You will also want to specify the client's needs (satisfactions and deficits) and developmental strengths and virtues. Conceptually, you need to understand what role the client's social network can play in helping him or her attain and maintain health as well as the possible barriers that these people might construct. You also need to know what potential the client has to mobilize energies for coping with stressors; that is, what strengths, virtues, and assets the client can build upon. Specific questions that relate to these resources are given in Table 10-4. Again, we have identified concepts and theoretical bases to be utilized in the analysis of data.

As you analyze the data within the context of the relevant concepts and theoretical bases, you will again make interpretations and diagnoses with intervention goals in mind. Your interpretive purpose will be to determine (a) the value attached to each component of the external social network (that is, family, friends, and health care providers) and (b) the nature and extent of the individual's internal resources.

Your diagnosis will specify the external and internal resource potential. Specifically, you will establish need satisfaction and deficits, keeping in mind each level of basic and growth needs, and you will specify your client's strengths and coping state. Your long-term intervention goal is to promote affiliated-individuation with as little ambivalence as possible, and thereby promote a dynamic, adaptive, and holistic state of health. These relationships among the interpretive purpose, diagnoses, and long-term intervention goals are given in Table 10-4.

GOALS AND LIFE TASKS

This final category has five major focuses for you to consider:

1. Your client's current goals
2. Your client's planned goals
3. The relationship between current and planned goals
4. The cognitive methods utilized
5. The relationship between chronological age and actual task resolution

As you plan interventions within this category you will note that some goals are directed toward satisfying basic-need deficits and that others are directed toward developmental task resolution. When clients are *impoverished*, they have such extensive basic-need deficits that they are generally first concerned with satisfying these deficits. This is often done by immediate, short-term goal attainment. It is difficult for these individuals to be concerned with long-term goals or resolution of developmental tasks. Therefore, our first concern is basic-need deficit resolution. Many small goals may be mutually set to accomplish need satisfaction.

The second major aspect of goal attainment is related to developmental task resolution. As you aggregate and analyze data within this category, you will find that E. Erikson and Piaget have provided valuable insights. You will be especially interested in your client's comments about his or her life across the developmental stages, how the client describes important times in his or her life (and how these relate to the developmental stages, strengths and virtues), what developmental tasks the client is working on now (what current goals are), and what goals the client has planned for the future. Specific questions, related concepts, and theoretical bases are given in Table 10-5.

TABLE 10-4   Resource Potential

| | Aggregation and Analysis | |
Data Category Focuses	Questions	Concepts and Theoretical Bases

1. External resources:
(a) Social network
	1.1 What relationship does the client have with the family?	Affiliated-
		    Individuation
		Lifetime growth:
		    basic needs

(b) Support system	1.2 Is the relationship "draining" or "invigorating"? 1.3 Is the family near by? 1.4 Is the family accessible in other ways? 1.5 Does the client have supportive friends? 1.6 Are they available? 1.7 What is the work/play situation?	
(c) Health care system	1.8 What is the client's perception of the health care system? 1.9 How does the client usually use the health care system? 1.10 What does the client think you can do to help?	Self-care: personal model
2. Internal resources: (a) Self-strengths	2.1 What are the client's perceived strengths?	Erikson's developmental strengths and virtues
	2.2 What strengths are identified by others?	Basic-need satisfactions
	2.3 What level of basic needs are unmet?	Growth-need satisfactions
	2.4 What level of growth needs are unmet?	

	Synthesis	
Interpretive Purpose	Diagnosis	Long-Term Intervention Goals
1. Determination of the nature of the external social network including: (a) The degree of support available (b) Whether or not network members permit and promote: Dependency Independency (c) Whether network members are invigorating or depleting (that is, restore or diminish resources)	External support system: Personal Health care system Affiliated– Individuation state	1. Promoting affiliated-individuation with the minimum of ambivalence possible
2. Determination of the individual's internal resources including: (a) Developmental virtues and strengths (b) Need satisfactions; need deficits	Internal strengths and virtues Need satisfactions and deficits	2. Promoting a dynamic, adaptive, and holistic state of health 3. Promoting and nurturing coping mechanisms that satisfy the basic needs and permit growth-need satisfaction

TABLE 10-4 (Continued)

Aggregation and Analysis		
Data Category Focuses	Questions	Concepts and Theoretical Bases
2. Internal resources (*continued*)		
(b) Adaptive potential: (1) Feeling states	**2.5** What "feeling" statements does the client make?	Adaptive potential: APAM
	2.6 Is the client expressing feelings of tense-anxiousness? Of sadness-depression? Of fatigue? Of active-happiness? Of hope for the future?	
	2.7 What is the client's pattern of feeling statements (current adaptive potential)?	
	2.8 Does the client relate any feelings to object loss?	
	2.9 Is it real, threatened, or perceived?	
	2.10 Does the client have a potential transitional object for attachment?	
(2) Physiological states	**2.11** What physiological-need satisfactions exist?	Dynamic holism
	2.12 What physiological-need deficits exist?	
	2.13 What potential exists for current mobilizing of resources?	Adaptive potential: APAM
	2.14 Is one subsystem (4) in jeopardy in order to support another?	

	Synthesis	
Interpretive Purpose	Diagnosis	Long-Term Intervention Goals
2. Determination of the individual's internal resources (*continued*)		**2.** (*repeated*)
(c) Current potential to mobilize resources	Adaptive potential state: *Arousal Equilibrium Impoverishment*	Promoting a dynamic, adaptive, and holistic state of health. Promoting and nurturing coping mechanisms that satisfy the basic needs and permit growth-need satisfaction

TABLE 10-5 Goals and Life Tasks

	Aggregation and Analysis	
Data Category Focuses	Questions	Concepts and Theoretical Bases
1. Current goals	1.1 What seems important to this client at this point in life?	Lifetime development:
	1.2 What does the client state that he or she is trying to do?	psychosocial stages
	1.3 Are goals related to basic-need deficits?	basic needs
	1.4 Are they related to developmental tasks?	
	1.5 Is there ambivalence about these goals?	
	1.6 Is the client enjoying this task (as opposed to being threatened)?	
	1.7 What stage in development does this goal or goals represent?	
	1.8 Is there distress secondary to the client's goals and those goals identified by other data sources?	
	1.9 Is there grieving related to the goals?	Affiliated-Individuation
2. Planned goals	2.1 What are the client's planned goals?	
	2.2 How do they relate to normal developmental tasks? Basic-need satisfaction? Object attachment?	Lifetime growth: basic needs
3. Relationship between current and planned goals	3.1 When asked to describe various stages of life, does the client describe resolution of developmental tasks? Unmet needs related to developmental tasks?	
	3.2 What stages do these current and planned goals represent?	
	3.3 Is there a growth and development pattern apparent?	

Synthesis		
Interpretive Purpose	Diagnoses	Long-Term Intervention Goal
Development of an understanding of your client's stage of development including:	Developmental task(s) resolved	Facilitating congruent actual and chronological developmental stages
(a) Resolved tasks	Current psychosocial stage	
(b) Current psychosocial tasks addressed	Current psychosocial task in progress	
(c) Assets and barriers related to task resolution	Assets Barriers	

TABLE 10-5 (Continued)

	Aggregation and Analysis	
Data Category Focuses	Questions	Concepts and Theoretical Bases
4. Cognitive methods utilized	4.1 What is your client's favorite or major form of conceptualizing? 4.2 What developmental stage of cognitive growth does this typically represent? 4.3 Is there a relationship between psychosocial developmental task (stage) and cognitive developmental stage?	Lifetime development cognitive stages
5. Relationship between chronological age and actual task resolution	5.1 Is the identified developmental stage congruent with that expected by chronology? 5.2 Is there conflict related to a discrepancy between chronological and identified developmental stage?	

Synthesis		
Interpretive Purpose	Diagnoses	Long-Term Intervention Goal
(d) Cognitive methods utilized (e) Congruency of current tasks addressed with chronological age	Major cognitive process utilized	Facilitating congruent actual and chronological development stages (*repeated*)

SUMMARY

In this chapter we have suggested that the analysis of information obtained from your client and other sources be completed separately for the four major categories of data: description of the situation, expectations, resource potential, and goals and life tasks. For each category we have presented the kinds of questions you will ask yourself, the theoretical bases you will use, and the interpretive purpose that will shape your development of diagnoses and long-term intervention goals.

NOTES

1. We distinguish the concepts aggregate, analyze, and synthesize from one another as follows:

to *aggregate:* to compile or gather together

to *analyze:*   to examine critically so as to bring out the essential elements

to *synthesize:* to integrate into a holistic unit

2. This means that a simple statement reflecting the client's view of his or her current state of affairs is necessary. For example: chronic angina related to continuous conflict with adolescent daughter.

3. "Positive" means that the individual's self-image and projection of self is growth-directed and within the context of the normal range of development, considering the client's current stage of development. Some people call this hope. We do not specify "hope" per se because our intent is broader than a feeling of "not hopeless." We perceive this state to include a sense of self-worth in addition to a projection of the "self" into the future. Dying persons can have a self-projection that is futuristic and positive even though they perceive that there is no chance to live. These individuals perceive that a part of them will go on—their work, their ideas, their love, etc. will be carried on by others. Many persons also project themselves into a life after death according to their specific beliefs.

4. When thinking about this question, the nurse will want to consider whether the client seems to be experiencing stressors or distressors in one subsystem that are resulting in stress in another. For example, is the client hypertensive while simultaneously expressing unmet safety-security needs (does the client feel that his or her job is in jeopardy or that he or she is getting too old to keep up at work)?

11

Nursing Interventions

OVERVIEW

Once you have aggregated data, analyzed it, synthesized it, and arrived at diagnoses, you will be ready to plan interventions. We believe that it is not possible to specify standardized interventions since each human is a unique individual who has modeled his or her world in his or her own way. But since humans are also alike in many ways, we can plan interventions within the guidelines of their similarities. These similarities are reflected in five major principles. Each principle has an associated *aim* for intervention. Therefore, nursing interventions can be standardized in terms of the *aims* of the interventions. Stated another way, nursing interventions can always be planned systematically if the nurse follows the *aims* of the interventions.

In the following pages we discuss each general aim in detail and give illustrations from our client contacts. With each discussion we include a table of interventions to give examples of how each general aim may be translated into specific nursing interventions.

AIMS FOR NURSING INTERVENTION

The five *aims* of nursing intervention are as follows:

1. Build trust
2. Promote client's positive orientation
3. Promote client's control
4. Affirm and promote client's strengths
5. Set mutual goals that are health directed.

These aims are embedded in the philosophy and theoretical bases we use in our nursing practice. Table 11-1 lists five principles pertaining to similarities among humans and attendant general aims for intervention. All interventions are planned and implemented within the context of the *modeling* and *role-modeling* paradigm. Table 11-2 shows how intervention goals, the five principles, and the aims for interventions interface. Figure 11-1 shows the relationship between the aims of interventions and Maslow's hierarchy of needs.

TABLE 11-1   Relationship of Human Similarity Principles and Aims for Intervention

Principle	Aim
1. The nursing process requires that a trusting and functional relationship exist between nurse and client.	Build trust.
2. Affiliated-individuation is dependent on the individual's perceiving that he or she is an acceptable, respectable, and worthwhile human being.	Promote client's positive orientation.
3. Human development is dependent on the individual's perceiving that he or she has some control over his or her life, while concurrently sensing a state of affiliation.	Promote client's control.
4. There is an innate drive toward holistic health that is facilitated by consistent and systematic nurturance.	Affirm and promote client's strengths.
5. Human growth is dependent on satisfaction of basic needs and facilitated by growth-need satisfaction.	Set mutual goals that are health-directed.

TABLE 11-2   Relationships among Intervention Goals,
Principles, and Aims for Intervention

Intervention Goal	Principle	Aim
1. Develop a trusting and functional relationship between yourself and your client.	The nursing process requires that a trusting and functional relationship exist between nurse and client.	Build trust.
2. Facilitate a self-projection that is futuristic and positive.	Affiliated-individuation is contingent on the individual's perceiving that he or she is an acceptable, respectable, and worthwhile human being.	Promote client's positive orientation.
3. Promote affiliated-individuation with the minimum degree of ambivalence possible.	Human development is dependent on the individual's perceiving that he or she has some control over life (while concurrently sensing a state of affiliation.	Promote client's control.
4. Promote a dynamic, adaptive, and holistic state of health.	There is an innate drive toward holistic health that is facilitated by consistent and systematic nurturance.	Affirm and promote client's strengths.
5. (a) Promote (and nurture) coping mechanisms that satisfy basic needs and permit growth-need satisfaction. (b) Facilitate congruent actual and chronological developmental stages.	Human growth is dependent on satisfaction of basic needs and is facilitated by growth-need satisfaction.	Set mutual goals that are health-directed.

It helps to design interventions more systematically by mentally "working up through" Maslow's hierarchy with each specific *aim* in mind. This can be done while simultaneously giving care. Of course, we do it deliberatively when preparing for follow-up client

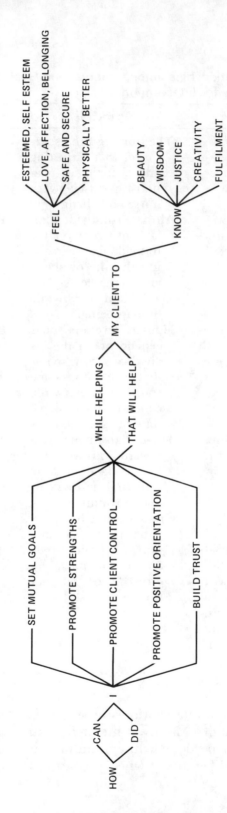

FIGURE 11-1 The aims of interventions and human needs

contacts. It becomes a part of our professional self-evaluation to do a systematic retrospective review of the same process. This also has heuristic value for further skill building and refinement. You might find it helpful to ask yourself the questions from Figure 11-1 while you plan experiences to meet your client's basic-need deficits and growth needs.

BUILDING TRUST

The nursing process requires that a trusting, interactive, and inter-personal relationship exist between nurse and client. In its simplest form, trust is developed with purposeful touch (holding hands, and so forth). Many nurses fear that the use of such simple interventions as these will result in a loss of respect for nurses and will lead to the demise of scientific foundations for practice. We would argue the contrary. That is, recognizing that these interventions are impor-tant, learning to explain why they are important, and studying the outcomes produced by their use will not only promote an ever-greater respect for nursing, but also provide a broader and more differentiated theory base for the practice of nursing. We are reminded of Thomas Huxley's and G. K. Chesterton's thoughts, respectively: "Science is nothing but organized common sense." "Nothing is so elusive as common sense."

One of the most effective ways of building trust is to listen well enough to understand a person's representation or model of the world. If we then demonstrate open, honest, direct, and kind behaviors in response, we are well on our way to inviting the "secure" attachment so vital to the well-being of many clients. Although most clients do not require that nurses be walking encyclopedias, or "perfect," or efficient, they do want their nurses to value and accept them for themselves. They always want some form of caring, even though some do not know how to ask directly for what will best connote that caring for them. Some want to be *cared for;* some want to be *taken care of;* others want both.

Secure attachments are characterized by a fundamental sense that the nurse is "on my side" *and* "capable of meeting my needs." It is a relaxed, comfortable feeling. Contrast secure attachment with "anxious attachment" in which dependency occurs but is mixed with a high level of anxiety. There is a constant threat of rejection. It is similar to the experience of a child who does not know what to expect from a significant care giver who is inconsistent, who alters approval with disapproval, acceptance with rejection, or scoldings with smiles. Such a child experiences conditional acceptance and receives a host of messages (both implicit and explicit) about "being good" or "not taking care of oneself." For clients whose psychosocial dynamics include incomplete basic trust formation, nurses may have opportunities unmatched by members of other professions for providing these clients with a "corrective emotional experience" associated with a secure attachment. This may be facilitated by the ongoing physically close contacts that are so natural to our practice with the ill and also compatible with well people's expectations of nurses.

There are a hundred small ways, natural to nursing, by which trust may be invited and fostered as we satisfy basic-need deficits. Note our list of examples relating to each level of Maslow's hierarchy of basic needs in Table 11-3. Other examples are dispersed throughout the pages that follow.

You will need to know what basic-need deficits exist if you are to focus your interventions on establishing trust. Remember that you must understand your client's model of the world before you can identify basic-need deficits. Purposeful nursing interventions to satisfy those needs will then incorporate your client's *self-care knowledge*. You may recall the care of the client in Chapter 9 in which a contract was used to keep the client "safe" in the nurse's absence. This intervention was designed for two reasons: the first was that this nurse (who had clearly demonstrated her concern for the client) had confidence in his ability to take care of himself; the second was to inform him that he had the control he needed to remain safe. Thus, the intervention helped build trust and simultaneously promoted client control.

When we identify in a client the unresolved task of trust, we place particular emphasis on creating conditions and interventions that facilitate the client in sensing a state of being taken care of and being cared for, feelings that are at the root of the development of trust. We have learned how extremely important this is if we want our clients to develop affiliated-individuation. This state comes only on the heels of a real sense of Eriksonian trust and autonomy.

In our work with persons with diabetes, it appears that a majority of those with juvenile-onset, insulin-dependent diabetes wanted and needed opportunities for working through basic trust issues. Of course, we encouraged decision-making too, for affiliated-individuation, not just affiliation, is our goal. We learned not to be surprised when clients wanted to be taken care of and frequently

TABLE 11-3 Building Trust

The following are examples only. Many are necessarily generalized for listing here. We invite creativity on the part of each individual nurse based on the client's model of the world. The first group of interventions applies in a general way to trust development. Those that follow pertain to each level of Maslow's hierarchy of basic needs.

General Guidelines

1. Give your name and identify yourself and your role clearly.
2. Make appointments for uninterrupted information gathering as client desires. *Keep* them. Establish time-delimited intervals for giving undivided attention and keep your word (or explain why you can't).
3. Invite expression of any questions, worries or concerns. Actively listen to elicit specific detail. Indicate that you remember information client has already given you.
4. *Sit down* to talk when you have time. Speak unhurriedly.
5. Maintain eye contact with occasional glances away (in general).
6. Convey "I accept you as you are," "It's not for me to judge," "I'm capable and willing," with mellow, low-to-medium voice tones, soft-lipped facial expressions, smiling eyes.
7. Listen when client speaks. Clarify what you don't understand. Admit, prn: "I still don't understand." "But I want to." "Try me again." If both you and client become frustrated, acknowledge that. Set another time to try again.
8. Dare to "bend rules" when it is important to client's peace of mind. Do it with attention to allaying apprehensions of other care givers. (Ideally *involve* them by sharing your theory base.)
9. Cheerfully fill all possible requests. When you can't, give your real reasons from a position of quiet strength and personal dignity. (Reasons may relate to client welfare, personal value conflict, institutional or system constraints, or personal reasons you prefer not to specify.)
10. If a value conflict arises between you and client, identify the conflict and do not withdraw from or reject client. Supply a substitute care giver if feasible or requested.
11. State the hour (or date) of termination. Give client prior notice of your departing. Introduce and channel trust to another care giver, as indicated.

While Meeting Biophysical Needs

1. Request permission for invasions of privacy and personal territory.
2. Invite full input of data when client identifies a physical concern.

TABLE 11-3 (Cont.)

If you are "too busy," set a time together for unhurried assessment and either keep the appointment or reset the time. Be honest about your time limitations. Share them in advance. Hold to them. Re-contract if necessary.

3. *Initiate* follow-up on earlier physical complaints. Evaluate *with* client the outcome of earlier interventions. Summarize "learnings" for each of you.

4. Accept client's report of physical discomforts without discounting or challenging them.

5. Use frequent fleeting touches to client's back and shoulders to decrease initial fear of closeness.

6. Remain with client when he or she is vomiting (dyspneic, chilling, having cardiac dysrhythmia). Verbally assure with "I will stay with you as long as you need me." Explore with client past experiences of such difficulties and measures that brought relief. Supply or build on these whenever possible.

7. Volunteer and spontaneously engage extra actions to increase comfort (bring pillows, drinks, diversions, etc.). Give back rubs.

8. Offer pain medications before client asks for them.

9. Stay with client after giving pain meds until client reports pain is subsiding. If you are unable to stay, offer to check back at designated short intervals and *do* it.

10. Answer call lights promptly and cheerfully.

11. Remain calm under pressure. (Use breathing techniques for yourself.) Sometimes share, "When I feel that way, I am often helped by breathing this way (demonstrate) (or thinking . . . , or having someone. . . .) This gives client permission to lean on someone or engage internal resources.

12. Allow client time needed to turn or move self. Do not rush client.

13. Handle wounds, wounded parts, aching, sensitive or painful body parts gently and slowly. Verbalize in advance: "I'll be gentle (as careful as possible). Tell me when you think I'm not." Commend clients when they do: "I'm glad you told me." "That's helpful information." "Go ahead and 'bawl me out.'" "Feel free to do or say anything that helps you feel better." "That's the way." "Say it louder." "You're important." "I'm glad you're taking care of yourself (. . . helping me take better care of you)."

14. Tell client you will make (hourly) rounds (walking, telephone, etc.) to be available to meet his or her new concerns (pain relief, restlessness, environmental changes, etc.). Follow through.

15. Arrange for favorite foods.

16. Supply extra fluids and foods when indicated. Directly and unhurriedly assist the *impoverished* client to consume them.

TABLE 11-3 (Cont.)

17. Welcome the family's attentiveness and concern. Encourage their bringing "goodies" and "treats" that are compatible with client's welfare. (Discourage items only when you are *sure* they will cause harm.)

18. Invite family to participate in physical care if client wishes it and if family members wish to and are able. (Gain client's permission before asking family.)

19. Handle equipment quietly and smoothly. (Do your preparatory "homework.") Supply and freely share your information and expertise with colleagues. Include client when client desires.

20. Specify in advance what you will be doing in physical care procedures. Encourage responses and expressions of feelings. Do not take these responses personally, discount them, or hastily seek to modify them.

21. Tell (truthfully) what may be expected during test procedures. Inform client about the sensations that may possibly be experienced. Encourage client to share his or her feelings after test(s).

22. Share physical examination findings you make as "raw data" without interpreting or diagnosing. In response to client's queries, *first* ask what he or she is thinking. Listen carefully to responses to hear the possible meaning of a finding to client.

23. Use touch, as client assents, during painful procedures.

24. Spontaneously supply "treats" (transitional objects), based on data received about kinds of things that give client good feelings, for example, pictures, favorite music, crafts, quotations, plants, flowers, poems, Bible verses, fragrances, outdoor walks, outings, etc.

25. Build client's capacity to imagine or visualize self *within* a happy or peaceful scene or setting (or hear favorite music, psalms, etc., inside own head.)

26. With sensory impaired clients, observe special requirements, such as:
    face-to-face speech
    louder voice volume
    lower voice tone
    preannounced entrances
    additional lighting
    verbalization of furniture arrangement

While Meeting Safety and Security Needs

1. Invite and commend client's input into all decision-making that concerns the client. If client is unable or unwilling to make a deci-

TABLE 11-3 (Cont.)

sion or if the client directly requests you to make a decision for him or her, ordinarily do it cheerfully. Share your rationale for the decision and your belief that it will not be long before the client will be making his or her own good decisions.

2. Use smiling eyes, touch, soft-lipped facial expressions to convey acceptance of the client "just as he or she is."

3. Calmly accept client's refusal or unreadiness to share information or "comply" with plans made for the client by others. Do not withdraw—emotionally or physically—even when you disagree with or dislike the client's choice. Convey acceptance of the client's own timing for change.

4. Invite expressions of feelings or sensations during procedures, such as dressing changes. Whenever possible, alter any of your actions that are causing unnecessary discomfort. Explain what you are doing and why.

5. Acknowledge your own temporary feelings of frustration, annoyance, fear, and so forth, from a position of strength and awareness of your power to change your feelings or control your actions while continuing to have them. Use "I" statements. Stay with client during strong expressions of feeling. If you are too uncomfortable, find someone who can stay with the client.

6. Teach client to use "I . . ." sentences by using them yourself.

7. Commend all direct requests for help made by client. Meet all possible requests. Simultaneously verbalize:
"We want you to feel safe."
"We will keep you from harming others or yourself."
"We will see that no one hurts you."

8. Initiate restoring of interaction after client expresses anger through verbal abuse or withdrawal. Do not punish by counterwithdrawing or scolding.

9. Stay with client while he or she engages in physical self-care. Do not deprive client of attachment satisfactions as he or she becomes more independent. (The client needs to initiate or suggest "separation.")

10. Make perception checks of what the client's body language means. "Your shaking hands suggest you may be feeling scared. Would I be right?" or "I'm wondering if the twitching of your ankle means that you're feeling worried (or upset, anxious) about something? Would it help to talk?"

11. Verbalize feelings that come naturally to you (and others) in connection with particular situations. For example, say, "If that happened, I'd probably feel _____." (This may give client permission to learn to know his or her feelings.)

TABLE 11-3 (Cont.)

12. Do not automatically defend the hospital or other health care professionals when client complains about them. Listen, reflect, clarify, summarize, and accept.
13. Be direct about your own needs (without expecting the client to meet them). Ask directly for assistance when *you* need it. This may give the client with "be strong" messages permission to imitate your example, to be taken care of, and so forth.
14. Establish routines that assure the client that you are predictable and accessible.
15. Demonstrate competence when using technical skills.

While Meeting Love and Belonging Needs

1. Use touch according to client's comfort level. If client pulls away, start with very light brushing of the back or shoulders while observing client's acceptance level.
2. Use the following phrases as appropriate:
"You're worth it."
"You're the whole point of our being here to help."
"We all feel that way sometimes."
"I want to help; I like helping you."
"How can I be most helpful to you?"
3. Apologize when you are genuinely responsible and genuinely sorry for a regrettable feature in your relationship. (Use this intervention sparingly.) Set new standards based on what the situation has taught you both.
4. Make spontaneous pop-visits or phone calls during which you express your desire to be of any possible help. Set suitable time limits at the outset and stick to them.
5. Periodically check on client through unsolicited and unexpected visits or phone calls. Say "I enjoy being with you and I enjoy talking with you."
6. Invite the client to call any time of day or night. Agree that if you are indisposed at the time, you will be honest and will set another mutually satisfactory time.

While Meeting Esteem and Self-Esteem Needs

1. Verbalize your genuine enjoyment and appreciation of client's talents, abilities, qualities, actions, and so forth. Be specific. "Mirror" them for the client so that he or she will become aware of the qualities he or she may not have recognized, have taken for granted, or downplayed.
2. Use gentle humor to laugh *with* the client and yourself.

TABLE 11-3 (Cont.)

---

3. Verbalize your own "imperfections" matter of factly and with continued evident self-appreciation. This facilitates the client indirectly to conclude that she can accept herself as *she* is.)

4. Assure client he is important enough to have your attention even if he's not "sick or suffering." Support, reinforce, and commend the client's open and direct requests for support, assistance, and so forth.

5. Say that you are interested in your client, not her gallbladder, but reassure her that you are concerned with her gallbladder if she is concerned with it.

---

asked us to make decisions for them. The difficulty with this situation is learning how to take care of clients while simultaneously encouraging their autonomy. We want them to perceive that safety comes with having a nurturing attachment figure, but without experiencing being controlled by that person.

Let's expand briefly on that thought. Many nurses have expressed concern that permitting and encouraging attachment will result in prolonged dependency. The word commonly used in this connection is *regression*. The trick is to teach individuals that they can have both dependency and independency simultaneously. Many people think that these characteristics represent opposite ends of a single continuum. We frequently tell people straightforwardly that this is not so, that these are two different kinds of needs shared by all humans. Further, all humans have a need for a balance between these two, and the balance is called affiliated-individuation.

We encourage people to think about these relationships and to give themselves permission to have time when they need and want to be dependent and when they need and want independence. We compare meeting our dependency needs to "getting our batteries charged." Once charged, we're ready to join the excitement of the everyday world. Without an occasional charge, we run out of energy. We tell clients to learn where they can "get a hug" without paying in return! We give them permission to ask us for nurturance in the form of hugs and touches, and we willingly respond to these requests.

We often share our philosophy with clients. We describe Maslow's hierarchy and Erikson's developmental stages, stating that all humans want to be the best possible persons that they can be but sometimes they have difficulty because their needs are not met. We describe the relationship between basic-need satisfaction and developmental task completion. We hasten to add that we feel that most parents want to be good parents and love their children very much but just don't quite know how to meet their children's needs all of the time. We feel that these comments help clients build trust because they send clear messages that we accept people as they are but we have hope that they can become what they want to be. These comments also imply that we don't need to get into a series of statements and disclosures about their parents and themselves (unless the individual wants to discuss such issues). These comments also suggest to our clients that their feelings were correct: while their parents may have loved them very much, it is possible to feel unloved. At the same time, it is comforting to them to know that their parents really did love them.

We often comment on the messages that are sent to us as children that result in our burying our feelings. Such messages as "be tough," "don't cry," "don't be angry," and "be strong" teach us to hide our feelings. While these feelings are real and much a part of us, our parents sent those messages with the best of intentions. The important point now is to uncover them to learn what they are and with what they are associated. Then we can relearn what they can do *for* us instead of against us. We encourage clients to think of feelings as *effective* or *ineffective* rather than good or bad. We comment that what was effective last year may no longer be helpful or effective, since we change constantly across the life span. We use the analogy of creeping and walking, stating that it is helpful for the infant to creep because it gets the infant around, but the adult may find it more useful to walk. We state that as we learn about our feelings we learn how to control and enjoy them rather than having them control us and make us unhappy.

The use of indirect statements such as in the last few comments has been an important intervention for us. These statements say to the individual:

1. You may learn about your feelings, or you may not. The choice is yours.
2. If you choose to learn about your feelings, you will learn to control them.
3. You will also learn to like and enjoy your feelings.
4. Therefore, you will not be unhappy because of your feelings.
5. Feelings will not make you do things you don't want to do.

These directions (which are not perceived as orders or commands because the individuals are not told to learn about their feelings or to identify their feelings) are helpful in promoting the hope that things will be better in the future. Hope, according to Erik Erikson, is a natural outcome of task resolution in the first stage of life.

We use many kinds of interventions in establishing trust. These interventions range from verbal statements about their self-worth to touches, smiles, and so forth. We give our clients permission to be dependent while encouraging them to grow and be independent at their own pace.

For those at other stages of development, building a trusting relationship also deals with independence needs. Some people who are working on the first developmental stage will literally return to a total care state for a short period of time. With encouragement, though, and given the conviction that their nurse cares about them and will care for them, they will follow their innate drive toward growth and development.

We recall a story a colleague told us that demonstrates this point well.

A client arrived at the postcardiac surgery step-down unit where he was assigned to our colleague for care. When she entered his room, she greeted him with "Good morning, how are you?" He immediately responded with "Will you wash my face?" Now this unit has a day-by-day protocol describing what post-op patients (note the word "patients") should be able to do for themselves, and patients are encouraged to do what is on this protocol list. Each patient is given this list and knows exactly what he or she is "expected" to do.

Our colleague, out of habit and socialization, immediately told her "patient" that by this time he should be able to wash his own face since it was on the step-by-step protocol. (We know this nurse. She is one of the kindest, gentlest women we know, and we are fairly certain her comments were made with much kindness. Nevertheless, this simple statement interfered with the establishment of a trusting relationship.)

The patient blew up in anger and told her to get out and not to come back. He didn't want to see her again. She went to the nurses' desk, thought it all over, and decided that he needed to be dependent before he could be independent. He was probably worried about how safe he was on this new unit. So she coura-geously returned to his room, apologized for the bad start, told him she cared about him and how they could work together. She asked if they could start over and told him that she would be happy to wash his face. She finished her story with the com-ment that by the end of the day he was doing everything he was supposed to do and without assistance. In fact, he was telling her she'd better come in and put her feet up because she must be tired. He not only was able to take care of himself but also had sufficient energy to take care of the nurse he had learned to trust because of her simple demonstration of acceptance and caring.

Individuals in autonomy need reassurance that the decisions they are making are "good" decisions and that they have "permis-sion" to make these decisions. They want to be reassured that the nurse will not reject them or discount them if their decision happens to be in conflict with that of the nurses or doctors. This is particularly important when we think about the possible incongruency in goals set by the various members of the health care team. We remember one woman who insisted on being allowed to leave the hospital for a few hours so that she could take her car in for repairs. Since she was only a few days post-op from major surgery, everyone was upset with her. She said that she was unhappy because her "favorite nurse" didn't understand how important it was to her to get her car fixed. Now, we realize that this may seem extreme, but our guess is that no one helped this woman think about other ways she could have gotten her car to the garage (a neighbor, a friend, perhaps a nurse). Instead, she was criticized and discounted for not following "orders." The staff reported that they didn't particularly like this woman be-cause she "wouldn't take care of herself." At the most fundamental level, though, she *was* taking care of herself.

How we establish trust depends on the developmental stage of the individual. In our experience, the higher the developmental task the individual is working on, the more likely the person will accept the nurse without difficulty. Since those working on initiative and higher levels have already completed the tasks of trust and autonomy (to some positive degree), they have a base of experience that has taught them they can depend on *being cared for and being taken care of* when they need it.

At this point we will clarify how we view the technical, hands-on skills of nurses and how we see those skills fitting into our scheme of developing trust. Since nursing means helping people take optimal care of themselves through interactive and interpersonal processes that promote growth, and since basic needs include physiological needs, we believe that technical skills are important to nursing as a vehicle for meeting basic needs. They are not, of course, the only means, but they certainly have their place. Skills and procedures performed for a client can be powerful tools for the speedy development of trust. From a dozen angles a nurse is given the opportunity to demonstrate caring: by gentleness of touch, voice, and facial expression; by considerations of client preferences; by eliciting feedback in order to follow every possible suggestion, that can be implemented; by offering various direct and indirect suggestions for the relief of pain; by supervised practice in relaxation skills; and the use of humor. Skills and procedures also present opportunities for subtle, compounded, and superimposed interventions that are intended simultaneously to meet unmet basic needs and to promote movement toward developmental task completion. A procedure as simple as bathing a client may be purposefully filled with constructive indirect suggestions designed by a creative nurse. How this happens will become more clear as we describe below some actual client situations. We applaud nurses in every setting who are developing the highest level of technical expertise of which they are capable. It is our hope that they will engage these skills and techniques as *tools* for the nurturance of self-care actions that promote optimum health.

We have tried to convey the belief that trust constitutes both being cared for and being taken care of in response to *perceived* needs. Very explicitly, *taking care of* a client is not sufficient for developing the type of trust we propose. Often, people learn that they can be taken care of (that is, lean on someone), but they are not certain that they are truly cared for, or accepted, as a human who is worthwhile, respectable, and important. We will expand on this concept when we talk about the client's positive orientation.

We have concentrated on factors involved in promoting trust in the client, but so far we have ignored the characteristics of the nurse as being important in this interpersonal process of nursing. We now turn to considering the importance of the nurse as an influencing factor. We believe that the nurse contributes extensively to the client's ability to develop a trusting relationship. Several authors have written about the helping relationship; we do not intend to duplicate their thoughts. But we would be negligent if we didn't include some of our observations.

Sometimes the nurse is tired and unable to be objective about a person's behaviors and attitudes. We need to keep in mind that we, too, are humans, with feelings, values, and old learnings that affect our current behaviors. We bring all of ourselves to our interactions with our clients. How many times have we heard the nurse say the following? "He reminds me of my dad." "He reminds me of a patient I once had who was really terrible." "Patients who take Bed C are always cranky."

Not only do we tend to identify clients with people we have known in the past, we also have a tendency to displace our own momentary feelings onto our clients. Take, for example, those times when we become irritated because we have just had a disagreement with a colleague (perhaps a communication sequence that felt "discounting") and then transfer such discounting onto our client. This, of course, will not be a major problem if it happens only once in a while, but if it becomes our pattern of communicating, we will have difficulty establishing trusting relationships with our clients. Trust is built on acceptance, not discounting. Table 11-4 lists attitudinal messages that the nurse conveys in developing trust.

One final point: Persons in a state of *impoverishment* are in great need of a trusting relationship with the nurse. This relationship helps them learn to feel "I can relax. I'll be OK. I'll be taken

TABLE 11-4   Attitudinal Messages the Nurse Can Convey When Developing Trust

You count.
I'm on your side.
You are valued for being you.
You have the right to be, to exist.
This world needs you—as you are.
You have a right to ask for and receive what you need.
You have a right to know your own feelings.
You have the power to make good decisions.
You can disagree with me and still have my respect and acceptance.
I will help you control your behaviors when you need help.
Your decisions can be made based on your thoughts, feelings, and experiences.
You are like your fellow human beings, but you are unique.
I enjoy your presence.

care of and cared for. I won't be rejected or abandoned if I behave badly or don't keep on my mask." In turn, these feelings free persons to use energies in attaining health rather then defending themselves, or fearing that they can't defend themselves. Nursing interventions for *impoverished* individuals are direct and are based on the assumption that individuals need to be cared for and about, that there is a reason for them to continue to *be*. Interventions for persons in the state of *arousal* are less direct. Indirect care is generally related to the drive for independence and attainment of control, while direct care generally relates to the need for dependency. If you are confused about these differences, picture the general type of care that an infant needs in order to survive and grow, as opposed to the care a toddler needs. Both infant and toddler need a little of each kind of care, just as both the *aroused* and *impoverished* need a little of both. But remember that there is an emphasis on one type of care over the other at each stage.

PROMOTING POSITIVE ORIENTATION

Promoting positive orientation has two aspects: The first aspect is to promote self-worth, the second is to promote hope for the future. These two perspectives go hand-in-glove, but also provide two different ways to think about necessary interventions. Both are related to our need for affiliated-individuation.

The issue of one's self-worth has been described in various ways in the literature. Some deal with the issue of self-image, and others talk about identity. We believe that self-worth can also be thought about in terms of the individual's worth, *simply because the individual is a human being*. This may sound strange, but we often have clients who cannot identify one single reason for being valued. We think that this occurs partly because our acceptance from others is often conditional, that is, acceptance is based on what we do, how we act, what we produce. We learn that unless we can do, act, and produce, we are not worthwhile. This can mean a great deal to people who suddenly find themselves confined to bed or chair. Interventions can be planned to promote a perspective of self-worth based on being unconditionally accepted. Take, for example, the man who refused to let his family visit him while he was dying, bedridden, incontinent, and emaciated. When asked what the problem was, he responded, "Who'd want to be with me? Look at me. I'm no good for anything." The nurse's responses addressed his worth. He was told that he still had much to offer his family; that his existence and his presence gave them a great sense of comfort; his family wanted to be near him; they wanted to share his life with him, not to talk or do anything, but *just be there*; this togetherness made them feel better. He was also reassured that he had the choice and did not have to have any visitors if he did not want them. He readily changed his mind about their visiting, allowed them to share with him the remainder of his life, including a peaceful death.

This problem of self-worth is also evident in those who are not hospitalized. Some people feel that no matter what they do, it would never be good enough. They must be perfect, and just when they approach perfection, their goal eludes them. The only way that they are acceptable human beings is when they are perfect. Sometimes these people develop a sense of helplessness or hopelessness. Frequently they keep trying but never quite feel good about what they accomplish. They never achieve more than a state of conditional acceptance. These individuals often demonstrate the Type A behavior described by Friedman and Roseman (1).

We include some examples of statements that we have found helpful with these individuals: "Thank you for being you." "I enjoy our interactions." "You are a special person." "The world is a better place to be in just because you have been here."

The intervention, "Thank you for being you," is sometimes followed by the client's asking the question, "What's so great about me?" If you choose to use this approach, be sure you have a ready answer. Some answers we have found useful have related to the *client's model* and strengths. "Your gentleness makes it a nice world to live in." "Your art adds beauty to the world." "Your smile brightens my day." "Your courage gives me strength." "Your love for life is delightful." "You *are*. That makes you special and important to me."

Another way to promote self-worth is to reassure individuals that they are like other human beings and that we value all people. A technique frequently used to assure people indirectly of our belief in their self-worth is to share our philosophy. We frequently start with a statement to the effect that we believe all people are important, worthwhile, and want to be the best that they possibly can be. We then go on to briefly describe Maslow's hierarchy, Erikson's developmental stages, and the affiliated-individuation concept. This technique was described in fuller detail when we talked about establishing a trusting relationship with individuals. While people are learning to trust, they frequently learn that they are worthwhile and count in our world. This sense of counting in a world that is so big, impersonal, and often difficult is sometimes hard to achieve. Nursing interventions designed to help people attain such a sense facilitate them in perceiving that there is a *future* and that they will be part of that future, whether they are alive or dead.

Sometimes development of this sense is enough to influence the difference between life and death. There are many recorded cases that suggest that a sense of "no future" has resulted in death. Take, for example, the study of Bantu witchcraft in which the medicine man says that the person will die, and he does (2). A firm belief that one will die seems to result in a physical response leading to cardiac arrest in these individuals. Others have reported that hopeless feelings from the loss of a loved one can be related to increased incidences of sickness and death (3).

Sometimes these individuals need what Jourard has called an "invitation to live" (4). Many times the nurse is the only one projecting a "future" for the client that is worth "fighting for." She can suggest that life is indeed worth living and worth the struggle. She can do this by demonstrating that there is someone who does care what happens. If a nurse can manage to sustain a client through a period of feeling "What's the use?" it may be possible for the client to emerge from his or her *impoverished* state to find his or her own reasons to live.

Positive expectations are sometimes best conveyed through deliberately phrased assumptions, such as when a person who is naturally scared he or she will die in surgery hears the nurse say, "I'll be here when you get back." This statement conveys the nurse's belief that the client will not die, he will return, and will continue to exist.

Often the *impoverished* person can be sustained by visits every half-hour, each one promised in advance, allowing for a passage of time. This intervention meets basic needs ranging from the level of safety and security to those of esteem. If during the visits the nurse touches or intervenes physically, needs at all levels are addressed.

Rekindling in people a sense of their own power to bring about some significant change also promotes hope and future expectations. Sometimes individuals feel so overwhelmed (*impoverished*) that they cannot believe they have the ability to change, to learn, to perform a new act. You can remind them that they have had greater mountains to climb in the past and have been able to climb them because they took them in small steps. For example, when they were three they couldn't read or write, or add or subtract or multiply or divide. (We purposefully make a long list like this so that we can point out strengths that they now have.) If at that age we had insisted they read the instructions for assembling a table, they could not possibly have done it. But now they can read the instructions and understand what all of the words mean. They know what the words "nut," "bolt," "leg," "top," and so forth all mean. They can read the instructions and follow them one step at a time until they have an assembled table. When they first saw the ABC's, they couldn't imagine what they meant, how to write them, say them, or place them in sequence. Now, however, all of that is so simple, just as what they are going to learn to do to change will seem so simple once they have learned it. Building on past accomplishments (strengths) to build a future will help your client improve self-worth and learn how to project himself or herself into the future.

While trying to help your clients perceive themselves as worthwhile and a part of the future, you will want to remember that sometimes *impoverished* persons have great difficulty mobilizing sufficient resources to deal with anything but the here and now. Projection into the future, for some, can be overwhelming, especially if they feel that all interactions *tax* them, rather than *energize* them. With these individuals it sometimes helps to make simple statements such as, "Right now you are probably too tired to think about this, but *soon* you might want to think about how we can work together to help you feel better. I know a lot of tricks that have worked for others; some of them might help you. When you feel like it, we can talk more about it."

Another way to handle *impoverishment* is to focus on the goal. Take, for instance, a post-op client who needs dressing changes that require the client to move and are uncomfortable. You can say something to the effect that you need to change the dressing and clean the wound to help the tissue get *healthier*. Together you can work out a way that will promote control by the client. You will want to ask the client: How do you think you can best help? How would you like to be rolled to the side? How would you like to be supported? What would you like to think about as you are having your dressing changed? Finally, you can say, "Each change helps your tissue get healthier and healthier, and soon it will be as strong as all of your other healthy tissues." Let us summarize with an example.

> The nurse was working with a 30-year-old woman who had been struggling for many months with whether or not she should give up her old maladaptive coping patterns to take on new, healthier patterns. When it appeared that the struggle was at a peak, it was gently suggested that she seemed to be between a rock and a hard place. She needed to give up old ways, or she might die. Yet the new ways seemed pretty scary. She commented that either way she faced death. If she continued with the current patterns, she would certainly die soon. However, giving them up meant the death of a part of her that provided safety and security. She wasn't sure she could survive without those coping patterns. Clearly, the decision to change was hard. The control for life and death was also hers. Education was no answer. She knew more about her particular illness than most patients in a similar position.

By *modeling* it seemed clear that her struggle was the same as that experienced when an individual moves through the stage of autonomy (5). This client needed support to be autonomous. When it was suggested that she might fear opening the box (of the future) because she thought she'd find worms inside, she admitted that was her fear. She was reassured that while this was possible, it seemed more likely that she would learn that what might look like worms were really caterpillars, caterpillars that would evolve into lovely butterflies if granted freedom, butterflies that would add beauty and joy to the world. The client made marked improvement from that point on.

Modeling your *client's world* is essential if you want to *role-model* a healthier, happier world for the client's future. Each human is uniquely different in how he or she has interacted with his or her world, met needs, resolved developmental tasks, and so forth. But each is like the others in that he or she *wants* his or her world to be good. As we strive for this better world for our clients, we need to *role-model* the possibilities of new ideas, excitement, and hope within the context of their reality. The butterflies mentioned above are a simple example of this. *Role-modeling* is more than setting a good example. It is helping the individual perceive himself or herself in a new role without experiencing threatening loss of the old. It requires helping the client consider stressors as a challenge (or self-fulfillment) instead of a threat to basic needs.

A final way to facilitate individuals in developing a position of future orientation is to teach them how to project themselves positively into the future. For example, if you have a client who enjoys going to the beach, you can encourage him to imagine himself at the beach enjoying the warm sun, drinking a cold soda, sharing company with someone he likes. You would also state that he can imagine himself doing these things next month (or next summer) and that, while he's having such a good time imagining this state, he might as well dream a little. What would he really like to have there on the beach with him? What would he think he could imagine in his wildest dreams? Finally, what could he possibly work toward?

Some people will respond with, "What for? What good will that do?" We've found that these individuals need to be reassured that it's OK to dream, to fantasize, to hope. They will have difficulty in long-term goals if they cannot have hope. A response that has worked for us is, "What harm does it do? And maybe it would be fun." On occasion, we have been told that dreams are a potential path to disappointment. On such occasions we reassess our *client's model* of the world, and alter our *role-modeling*. If it is within the client's world that dreams always result in disappointments (perhaps because the expectations are too great, too grandiose), then it might be a good idea to *role-model* a less ambitious dream that can be developed and realized. Sometimes success comes in small steps. With such persons, a simple, specific, and very concrete goal that can be measured and achieved helps. Upon achievement, reinforcement (that the goal was achieved, that it felt good when it was achieved, and that it was possible to set goals and work toward them) helps clients learn that they can project themselves into the future and that they can make it work for them, not against them.

Table 11-5 lists other suggestions for promoting a positive orientation. As you review these suggestions and reflect on suggestions for the other aims of interventions, you will note that many interventions can be used for more than one aim. You will also think of many interventions you have used that are not listed. In both cases, this is as it should be. When you work with holistic people, it is expected that nursing will be both simple and complex. For example, the important communication skill of listening could easily meet the aims of trust, control, and positive orientation. Nat-

TABLE 11-5 Promoting Positive Orientation

Below are examples of ways by which a positive orientation may be promoted. Use your own creativity in modifying them and designing others based on your client's unique model of the world.

General Guidelines

1. Share personal philosophy—all human beings are important and worthwhile.
2. Reassure that the client is important because he or she *is*. Say that you believe all people are worthwhile and have something to contribute, no matter what their state might be.
3. Base many of your questions and comments on an implied future: "It won't be long before you'll...." "How long will it be before...?" "People like you don't usually take any longer than they need (in order) to...."
4. Respect and compliment client's full and free expression of dissatisfactions and concerns. "... can't begin to *solve* problems until they've first been identified."
5. Avoid any negative comments about client's condition, especially when client is not maintaining an active, assertive dialog with you and others. (Client may misinterpret and think that he or she has professional validation for despair and continued loss of hope.)
6. Use metaphors suggesting future growth and improved states of function: caterpillar to butterfly; clouds to sunshine; storms to rainbows; shadows and light to produce beautiful portraits.

When Meeting Biophysical Needs

1. Verbalize, "I'll be waiting for you when you get back," to the person who is going off to surgery.
2. Teach post-op deep breathing and coughing before the person goes to surgery.
3. Reassure client that you will stand by to give all possible pain relief (for example, to post-op and terminally ill persons).
4. Facilitate contact with people who have undergone similar experiences and still enjoy meaningful lives.
5. Check in frequently with a critically ill client. Say you'll return and set short time intervals between checks. Say: "We will do everything there is to do. We will not leave you alone. We care."
6. Report to client every physical gain, however small, using quantities and rating scales whenever possible. Summarize gains and achievements periodically.
7. Encourage client to identify any symptom-free or "successful"

TABLE 11-5 (Cont.)

time periods. Explore these for common characteristics. Suggest to client that these periods "hold the key" (are important data) to an eventual symptom-free or controlled state.

8. Explain the current theories on the effect of positive feelings on positive physiological outcomes and negative feelings on negative physiological outcomes. The client *can* act to replace negative with positive feelings; therefore, optimism can be appropriate.

9. Ask client or support system to identify things and people that give the client good feelings. Provide or enlist or engage them.

While Meeting Safety and Security Needs

1. Counsel "slow but sure is often best" (as means of consolidating gains).

2. Teach constructive ways of dealing with "catastrophic expectations."

3. Verbalize: "You may decide to give up an unhelpful behavior (symptom) just as soon as you can substitute a more desirable one (from your perspective) in its stead."

4. Refute the myth that infancy is a time of complete helplessness (6). Point out ways in which children make their needs known.

5. When client blames himself or herself for the current state of affairs, teach reframing by drawing the logical conclusion that the client can also *reverse* what he or she has "set into motion"; explain that the responsibility to "create" implies the ability to "undo."

6. Assist client in differentiating between his or her feelings and thoughts. Point out the common English idiom of "I feel . . ." wherein one ends sentences with a *thought* instead of verbalizing a *feeling* in the major categories of sad, glad, mad, or scared.

7. Reinforce that feelings can be client-controlled just as are thoughts and behaviors—that they can be "taken care of" in order to gain desired outcomes. For example:
   (a) Use feelings as *information* for problem solving, thereby *valuing* each feeling.
   (b) Replace unwanted feelings with those the client would rather have by choosing to "reframe" events that precipitate them, for example, seeing heelmarks on the kitchen floor as signs of active, healthy, loving family rather than as more work; hearing snoring of spouse as reassurance of spouse's continuing, valued presence in the family system; feeling scolding of parents as evidence of their love and caring, not their rejection;

TABLE 11-5 (Cont.)

hearing arguing of children as the promise of assertive maturity behaviors, not deliberate antagonizing of parents.

(c) Enjoy feelings as providing color and energy for living.

(d) Decide "how long" one will indulge or hang onto an unconstructive feeling ("rant and rave" for five full minutes; be sad until birthday).

(e) Defuse and becalm feelings nonverbally, as in vigorous motor activity.

(f) Deliberately use high-intensity feelings to "imprint" desired new messages about taking better care of self, liking self, and so forth.

(g) Verbalize feelings directly to another with sensitivity and expressed commitment to a desired outcome of mutual benefit.

8. When client requests it, pray with client when you can do so comfortably (or gracefully procure someone who will). Ask client for prayer's content.

9. Call in pastor, priest, or rabbi as client indicates.

While Meeting Love and Belonging Needs

1. Verbally express ideas, such as, "We're all in this together. You have your input and I have mine. Both of us desire that you should get what you need and feel cared for throughout this experience (no matter what the final outcome). I intend to see that that happens."

2. Point out potential reasons for client to "go on living."

3. Identify a specific or practical contribution the client is making or will be making to the family and members of his or her social network.

4. Report messages, calls, and inquiries of social support system members promptly and completely.

While Meeting Esteem and Self-Esteem Needs

1. Teach about unused potential throughout the developmental stages of life. Teach the value of learning how to stay healthy, and *get even healthier.*

2. Combat myths about old age, such as inevitable mental decline, much reduced or absent sexual function. Share the results of the latest research.

3. Point out specifically how and what the client has taught you (and others that you know) about people, life, ways of helping, and so forth.

TABLE 11-5 (Cont.)

4. Teach selected behavior modification principles that the client can apply personally.
5. Encourage client to enroll in classes to learn new skills, develop new interests, and pursue long-neglected ambitions or goals that are realistically still available (an 80-year-old could *still* learn to play the piano).
6. Encourage client to make a list of 30 inexpensive pleasures to put into action when the client is feeling low, and to keep this list conspicuously posted.
7. Encourage client's inventiveness and creativity and willingness to try out new experiences and to choose to break old, no longer useful "rules."
8. Reinforce that learnings from this experience, however, difficult, will be useful not only to the client but also to others in the future.
9. Identify client's past contributions to his or her social network and/or community. Allude to the unfinished aspects of the work still ahead.
10. Solicit client's opinion on ideas and projects for the future. Affirm your or others' dependence on the client for continued contributions that only the client can make.
11. Mutually design short, easily completed tasks requiring client's input for successful completion.
12. Remind client of the hope-giving aspects of his or her own expressed spiritual convictions and learnings, for example, steadfast love of God, forgiveness, adoption as sons and daughters, "all things work together for good," "The Lord is my Shepherd (Fortress, Rock, Help, Strength, Shelter, Shield, Defender, Light, Provider, Counselor, Guide, Comforter)."
13. Say that you enjoy working with your client.

urally, since each client is unique and has his or her own model, you will need to be creative. The whole point is that you can do what you do well and learn to be systematic and purposeful at the same time.

PROMOTING CLIENT CONTROL

Human development is dependent on individuals' perceiving that they have some control over their lives. The concept of client control is not a new one for most nurses. We have been emphasizing the need to educate our clients so that they will have more personal control. We have talked about involving them in planning their care. Nurses in intensive care units teach clients how to cough, deep-breathe, exercise, and perform other self-care measures. Nevertheless, many clients still don't *perceive* that they have control over their environment or their lives.

The concept of control that we promote is a much more basic process than simply teaching people techniques so that they can do something when we want them to. We are talking about the type of control needed if true affiliated-individuation is to be promoted. For example, the woman who insisted on having a sitter help her get well was one who was given our version of control. This woman had no desire to learn, to care for herself, to bathe herself, even to feed herself. She wanted total dependency (affiliation). Meeting her basic needs gave her a sense of control.

Too often, nurses think that the more control their clients have, the less they will have to do for the clients. Or, conversely, the more control the clients have, the more their clients will manipulate them. We feel that the manner in which control behaviors are acted out will be determined by the stage of development the individuals are working through. Adults may fluctuate among types of control needed, depending on how well their basic needs are met. Take, for example, the client described in the previous section who moved from wanting his nurse to wash his face (dependency) to the point where he was taking care of her (independence). Both are examples of client control.

Interventions designed to facilitate the client in perceiving control are most effective when they are designed within the framework of the client's model, within the context of the client's basic-need deficits and developmental stage. Sometimes nurses become confused about their clients' needs. Just as they think they have managed to understand a client, the client's needs seem to change. This is because humans grow and develop over time, and sometimes growth occurs very rapidly.

We recall one client who had become a problem patient.

She was being ignored and avoided as much as possible. Finally, in order to get her needs met, she threw her tray at one of the aides, yelling that no one cared about her, no one believed her, and she might as well be dead. A nurse consultant was asked what to do. The solution was fairly simple once the data were considered. This person felt unloved, uncared for, uncared about. The nurses thought that she was capable of taking care of herself, that there was really nothing wrong with her, and that she was just a manipulating, difficult person. Together with the assistance of the nurse consultant, the nurse and client shared their perspectives, each gaining new insights. The nurse agreed that her client probably felt unloved, uncared for, and uncared about, and then stated that she (the nurse) really did care about her and really did want to help her. The nurse also stated that she simply hadn't known what to do (short of "specialing" her) to change the situation. After this exchange, the client was able to articulate that she would feel safer, less isolated, and abandoned if she knew the nurse would stop in to see her on a regular basis. This seemed fairly simple, so they agreed that the nurse would be in every hour to simply check on her client. This seemed to resolve the problem.

You will note that with these interactions the nurse aimed to develop both trust and control in the same intervention. Another way to handle a similar situation, one in which the client is "constantly on her call light," which usually results in nurses ignoring her request to meet basic needs, would be to write a contract with the client. The nurse would promise to answer the light within 15 minutes (or within ten minutes or five minutes—whichever would make the client feel safe and cared about) and would spend five minutes with the client *if* the client, in turn, would try to call no more often than necessary. We have found that when we do this, we are tested initially; but if we keep our end of the bargain, the client almost always does too. The point is that people are innately driven toward a state of affiliated-individuation, depending on how well their needs are satisfied. When they sense that we really care about them by giving them control over how their needs will be met and which needs are to be met, then these individuals' basic needs are often met without further interventions. The desire to belong and give to others emerges, and the nurse is often the recipient of this innate drive.

We remember one young girl who was dying of cancer.

Her abdomen was painfully bloated, her buttocks leaked serum from constant pain injections, and her hair was almost all gone.

The nurses felt bad for this girl and tried to *take care of her*. They brought her gifts, sneaked in foods that were forbidden (hoping that she would eat *something*), and showed many other kind and interested gestures. Nevertheless, she seemed to eat less, became less and less responsive (although her physical condition didn't really warrant a nonresponsive state), and cried more frequently. The nurses were fearful that she wouldn't get a chance to go home, which she had wanted to do. One evening one of the nurses, in desperation, asked this client/patient what would make her feel better (7). "All I need is my dog. He makes me feel good—he's so soft and cuddly and cute. That's all I need. But I know that we can't have dogs in the hospital. I've already asked the nurse on days." The evening nurse thought the situation over and decided that a "cute cuddly little dog"—probably just what this girl needed—couldn't possibly be all that bad. So the nurse and mother agreed: tomorrow evening when the same nurse was on duty, mom would bring in the dog. He was so small he could be brought in a bag and no one would ever know. That evening the girl asked for food, the first in several days. The following evening, right on target, mom and "cute, cuddly dog" arrived. He was immediately put under the covers, because that's where he stayed at home when they were in bed. The girl and nurse both agreed that it might be better if the doctors didn't know, for they might not understand. When the doctors made their rounds they never suspected that "cute, cuddly dog" was in the girl's bed, keeping her "warm inside," making her feel important, valued, and loved. The client improved rapidly, developed a delightful sense of humor (that no one had suspected she possessed), and went home for the remaining six months of her short life.

Control comes in many forms. Consider another case:

One day, while walking down the hall of a medical-surgical unit, a nurse heard a strange sing-song sound coming from a room. Peering into the dark interior she saw a solitary woman in her late forties lying flat on her bed chanting. She entered the room and asked the client to tell her about herself. "Is there anything you would like to tell me? I'd like to know you better." The story unfolded. The woman had had terrible headaches, headaches that came out of the wall of her room, traveled up her foot, circled wildly in her abdomen, shot up through her body, and landed in her head. She had been sent to the hospital for a checkup. Her doctor suspected she had a brain tumor or some other pathological problem.

The woman continued with her story. She had been in a Polish concentration camp. Her parents had died there, and she had been "forced to walk on their bodies," an experience that made her feel that she was taking in their lives through her feet. She had been raped by a prison guard, became pregnant, and underwent an abortion. The abortion, she said, touching her abdomen where the pain circled and circled, had been an "awful" thing. She had been fairly well until a few months ago when her headaches first came on her.

Listening to this woman's story, the nurse realized that there were some serious guilt problems that needed to be dealt with, but that due to the nature of the woman's hospital admission and the other constraints of the immediate environment, such needs should be addressed outside the institution. Nonetheless, it seemed appropriate for the nurse to *role-model* a slightly healthier world for this woman *now*, for she had bad headaches that *did need* to be controlled. The nurse still needed more data about this client's self-care knowledge before she could *role-model*, however. Thus, she asked if the woman felt she *needed* to have her headaches. The immediate response was, "Oh, yes, dearie. I thought about giving them to the ambulance driver—he hit every bump just so it would make my head hurt even more—but then I decided that wasn't really fair. Besides, I need them. They're mine."

The nurse, now *role-modeling*, agreed emphatically that the headaches were indeed hers, and that no one else had a right to them, nor did she probably want to give them *all* away. But, she wondered, did the woman need them all day long? They seemed so debilitating. Maybe if she didn't have them all day, she could enjoy life just a little more. The client agreed. She missed her garden, missed being with her children and grandchildren. "But what can I do?"

The answer seemed simple. The woman needed the headaches, but only sometimes, not all the time. When you have something you don't really need all the time, but are fearful of having it out of your sight for fear of losing it, you keep it nearby, though not necessarily in or on you (*modeling*). So the nurse blocked out a square in the bulletin board at the foot of her client's bed, suggested that this was a good, safe place that she could keep an eye on, and that the client would probably want to keep her headaches there most of the time. It was suggested that they could stay there safely for 23 hours each day (*role-modeling*), but that the woman might take them back for an hour each day just because she needed them (*modeling*). The client was delighted: a perfect solution.

Over the next several days the woman underwent several tests, many of which were very painful. Nevertheless, her head-aches appeared only in the evening between five and seven o'clock (about the same time of day that her parents had died). All her tests were returned negative, and the woman was prepared for discharge to her home. She was somehow in better shape than when she had arrived, but no one (except the woman herself and this nurse) knew why.

On the day of the discharge the client became markedly agitated. She insisted on seeing the nurse who had helped her with her headaches. What was she to do, she wanted to know. The doctors were perplexed, advised her to keep taking her pills, and shrugged their shoulders. Her nurse, knowing what the problem was, told her not to worry, got an envelope, and wrote "headaches" on the front of it. She told the client to put her head-aches in there and take them home with her. And the client did.

Control comes in strange forms, but invariably it requires that we listen attentively to what our clients tell us about *their worlds*. We can make suggestions, as in this example in which the outcome is healthier than the preceding state, but we must always remember that it is the client who finally has control. It is the client's body, mind, and soul that we are talking about.

Control can be given to seemingly comatose people. There is one case of an individual who was very, very ill. It seemed that this person was not responding to stimuli; she had been in intensive care for a period of time. Placing the client's hand on her own chest, the nurse said quite simply, "You are alive and breathing very well. Can you feel those nice strong breaths? Can you feel your chest go up and down? You are making it do that. You have control over your breath-ing and your chest going up and down. You can make it go faster and you can make it go slower. You have strong respirations. Soon you will have more control over other parts of your body, too. Only you know which parts of your body you can control, but soon you will have more control."

Within these statements were several messages: You are strong. You have control. You'll have more control. You know you have control, and you know what you control. The nurse *modeled* her client's world, identified a strength, promoted control, and encouraged her client to expand that control to other parts of the body when the client was ready.

The client lived to tell the story, and stated that it was like an awakening for her. She had felt helpless and hopeless until she learned that she could make her breathing go faster or slower. That gave her strength to keep fighting. Control is as simple a thing as "When do you want your bath?" It can be as complex as that in the case just described. Table 11-6 lists several other examples of providing control.

TABLE 11-6 Promoting Control

Below are examples of ways in which control may be promoted. We encourage you to find ways particularized to your clients by which you might creatively meet this general aim.

General Guidelines

1. Inquire by what name the client prefers to be called.
2. Ask the simple questions: "What do you think causes this?" "What do you think you can do to help yourself?" "How can I help you?" Subsequent dialog may include offering more information, health principles, and so forth. *Listen again.* Take client's words *seriously* unless client is *obviously* kidding. (Remember that some kidding contains important truths.) Shape your responses in terms of the client's model of the world.
3. Ask the client what he or she needs to feel safe (safer) in specific situations that might arise. Then *do* or provide what you're capable of, for example, hold the client, sing or read to (or with) the client, pray with the client, provide information, or facilitate contact with others who may be able to offer safety by their information or presence [physician, significant others, important symbols, objects (pictures, prayers, pets)].
4. With *impoverished* persons, use information gained through observation or conversation with relatives, etc., to anticipate and supply unrequested objects similar to those in guideline 3.
5. Reinforce the idea that no decision is final: "You can change things

TABLE 11-6 (Cont.)

if you choose." "You have important data inside yourself that is available to no one else." "You are the best person to make final decisions after we tell you what we know, including health principles and objective observations and lab data that are external to you and less accessible to you. We will not reject you, whatever you decide. Ultimately, you're in charge."

6. Convey this concept: "Listening to your body's messages improves your skills at meeting your needs. It is mature behavior to ask directly for help when you need it." (Increased or developed responsiveness to "body messages" may be viewed as an early-warning *protective* capacity rather than causes for hypochondrical worries.)

7. Encourage client gently and tactfully to check out his or her "mind-reading" of others and unvalidated interpretations of others' nonverbal behaviors. (Using yourself as an example sometimes makes this easier. For example, say, "I've learned that if I think people are mad at me because of their tone of voice, it's helpful to check it out by asking them directly. Sometimes, I've been surprised to learn that they are fearful instead—or at least annoyed with something or someone else and not with me.")

8. Encourage client's expression of the "what if's . . ." that he is thinking about. Turn control back by asking, "If it should happen, how do you prefer we handle it?" (Do precrisis, anticipatory planning together.)

When Meeting Biophysical Needs

1. Let the client choose the time for the bath. Delimit or supply the time framework (as between 10 A.M. and 2 P.M.) *only* if necessary.

2. Follow *every* suggestion the client gives you about dressing (or -ostomy) changes as long as you do not feel you are compromising infection control or healing potential or your own peace of mind in terms of inordinate demands on your time. If this happens, *give* your real reason for declining the client's suggestions—courteously.

3. Let the person decide when to cough, deep-breathe, and so on, *before* or *after* receiving pain medication (share current theories beforehand, perhaps). Give ongoing feedback about the level of fluid in the lungs. Reinforce the sharing of responsibility for post-op anticomplication activities.

4. Ask client where she'd like injection given and what position she prefers for receiving it.

5. Invite a *nonimpoverished* client to participate in keeping track

TABLE 11-6 (Cont.)

of own intake and output, watching own intravenous infusion, and so forth. (Never pressure or require this.)

6. Explore what helped relieve nausea, dyspnea, pain, constipation, or arrhythmias in the past. Provide or encourage the same or similar measures. Be willing to try unconventional relief measures so long as they are not *known* to be harmful.

7. Teach overlapping of representational systems for symptom relief (8).

8. Share the observations you are making about color, pulse, respirations, and so forth. Be sure the client has this information (just as you have it) to enable client to participate fully in wise decision making (for example, when to stop walking and rest the first time after surgery, when to return to work). Give the client principles and information that the client needs to combine with objective and subjective personal data (including subjective material that may not have been expressed and what is known by the client at an unconscious level only).

9. Gain the client's perception of the strength of a symptom in quantitative terms. "On a scale of one to ten (worst possible pain), how would you rate your discomfort now?" Or, "How would you rate the pinkness of your urine (10 = blood red, 1 = clear yellow)?" "What was it (last time, yesterday)?" "Then what conclusions might you draw?"

10. Incorporate the client in deciding what dosages are needed for pain relief when sliding scales are in order. Obtain the client's numerical ratings of his or her pain from before and after the last dose of analgesic. Compare these with the rating client gives the current pain. Give client relevant principles of safe, effective pain relief and let client help decide whether more, less, or same amount will best help gain relief and still keep respiratory function, sufficient mobility, self-desired or required alertness, etc.

When Meeting Safety and Security Needs

1. Ask client what he or she needs from you to feel safe. Provide it. For example, the client will come to ask for pain medication at the first "twinge" to prevent delays that let pain mount to the level at which relief is more difficult to obtain.

2. Encourage and commend all questions and use of the call lights. "I'll be happy if what leads you to call turns out to be nothing." "No question or concern is foolish."

3. When client voices catastrophic expectations, teach client to ask,

TABLE 11-6 (Cont.)

"What's the worst possible thing that could happen? What control do I have over that worst possible thing?"

4. Teach negotiating skills: "You can ask directly (and kindly) for what you want and need. I will tell you my need also. Then we can decide together how things can be done so that both of us get most of what we need or want."

5. Set a framework of safety limits when client's safety is at stake. Honestly explain to client the reason for these limits. Within these limits, give full decision-making power to client. Avoid imposing your personal model, preference, or ideas. (Example: Client must take no longer than five minutes soaking off a burn dressing so as to prevent exponential increase in bacterial count. Does client wish to remove the dressing by self within that time limit or have nurse do it?)

6. Establish and hold to routines that client expressly desires and finds comfortable.

7. Teach relaxation skills, breathing techniques, and imagery to facilitate the client's perception of his or her ability to control the scary aspects of his or her experiences.

8. Teach the client to ask himself or herself what benefit or gain is associated with a particular habit or (maladaptive) behavior that the client wants to change. Explore the possible alternate ways of supplying those gains or advantages without the client's continuing to disadvantage or harm himself or herself.

9. Write things down for "visual learners" or "visualizers." Say them aloud in simple, repetitive formulas for those who are auditory, for example, "You have the power to change (when you are ready to)." "You have the power to take charge of your life."

When Meeting Love and Belonging Needs

1. Verbalize your willingness to be with the client even when client has no immediate "obvious" discomfort or suffering. Encourage client to ask openly if he or she wants companionship during meals; expressions of commendation, approval, or support from nurse; reminders of strengths. Grant the request along with praise for "asking directly for what you need and want."

2. Verbalize your interest in the *client:* "I'm 'pulling for you' in this plan. I want to know how you're doing. How often should I check back?"

3. Follow client's request for dependency when it is used as a "test" of being cared for. (This gives the client control through being taken care of and sets the stage for movement toward independence.)

TABLE 11-6 (Cont.)

4. Invite client to call any hour of day or night for encouragement, help, or support. Establish in advance that you will always be honest and if you cannot talk or be available at the moment, you will arrange a mutually suitable alternative time. (Having offered this option to many clients, we have never had this abused.)

5. Express, "Let's keep in close touch this week. Shall I telephone you, or you me?"

6. Help the client attend to what actions and/or objects from others bring about good feelings. Support the client in identifying people who will be able and willing to meet a current need on request. Support the client's directly, kindly asking for what client needs. Verbalize that it's healthy and good to ask people you trust for time, attention, support, hugs, and so forth. Also teach that if the first one(s) asked cannot comply, there are others who will be able and willing. *Be* one of those to the client if necessary while exploring how the client may build or increase a support system from the existing social network.

7. Give preframed choices, such as, "Shall we share this information (event) first with your father or your mother?" (*Sharing* the information is not a choice.)

8. Ask, "Who would you like to be included in this teaching session (use of glucagon in emergencies, how to inject)?" (There *will be* a teaching session.)

When Meeting Esteem and Self-Esteem Needs

1. Explore what would help client to feel good about self. (Answers may vary as widely as the number of clients you contact.) Support the client in reaching out for achievable things, persons, or events. *Now*, while you stand by. Summarize the client's accomplishment(s) when completed.

2. Help the client to think of feelings as neither good nor bad, but as information to be used to help make good choices for himself or herself. For example, if client is jealous, what of? What does client need to feel less threatened? Can client take steps to develop abilities, skills. What might stop the client? When will client begin? (Well begun is half done.) Use a transactional analysis framework to help client understand communication patterns (9).

3. Convey the idea that tears were designed for a purpose. Suggest that the client might be grateful they flow freely.

4. Encourage and assist client to choose to do kind, thoughtful things for others. "It's good to take care of yourself *and* of others, too." (This is not for the *impoverished* client.)

TABLE 11-6   (Cont.)

5. Help client to be as supportive and kind to self as he or she knows how to be to others. (Some initially respond to ". . . so you will continue to have ability and energy to be kind to others.")
6. Summarize self-care accomplishments: "Are you *aware* of how skillfully you are managing your dressing changes (new life style, work situation)?

In either case, it's all control. If we are to utilize these concepts in conjunction with patient education, it might help to review Maslow's ideas about learning: People are both afraid to learn and eager to learn. We need to *model* our clients' world before we force knowledge on them, if we are to promote their control.

We now turn our attention to the nurse as a member of the team that promotes client control in health care. As stated earlier, nurses will want to think about themselves, their philosophy, their expectations for clients and client care as they decide whether or not the concepts presented here are compatible with their own personal style. Sometimes nurses get into "one-upsmanship" positions when working with people. Probably this happens for a variety of reasons, including the fact that nurses often perceive themselves in "one-downmanship" positions and so, with unmet esteem needs, turn on their clients. We propose that it is helpful for you to think about your perspective on control issues so that you can determine whether or not you would be able to promote control as described in this section.

We have found Karpman's game triangle from transactional analysis theory a help in the analysis of interactions in one-up and one-down situations (10). In the practice of nursing, the client and nurse ideally have an open, honest, direct, and kind relationship wherein needs and desires may be freely discussed and limits can be set by mutual agreement. The key lies in the concept of *holism*, for in interactive and interpersonal relationships both the nurse's and the client's needs are at stake. Nurses who need to control their environment, including the people in it, rather than understand and work with it, may have difficulty promoting control in clients.

The nurse's goals and expectations for her client must also be considered in the promotion of client control. Sometimes the nurse has to sort out who she works for, what her goals are, and what she expects to have happen before she can be concerned with the promotion of client control. Nurses often feel so constrained by legal and bureaucratic powers that they assume that they have no choice but to take control over their clients rather than promoting it in them. We contend, however, that the nurse can be both safe and promote client control. Let us give you two examples.

The client had been confused and getting out of bed frequently on an evening shift. He pleaded not to be restrained and promised not to get out of bed anymore. He insisted he was no longer confused. The midnight nurse was in conflict. She empathized with her client; it must be a horrible feeling to be tied down. She also knew that she and the hospital were liable if her client should fall. The nurse honestly and kindly shared her dilemma with the client. "I feel uneasy about your earlier confusion and the wandering you have been doing. I don't know whether it is due to your medicines or not. I know how much you hate being tied down, but I cannot take a chance. In your present state you might try to get up and then fall. I am responsible for your safety while you are in the hospital. Here's something we might try that will make us both happy." The following compromise was cheerfully accepted by the client. The nurse would, at his suggestion, check him hourly to ask orientation questions which would allow him to demonstrate his clarity of mind to her satisfaction. Halfway through the night, a reevaluation of their mutual decision would take place. What was the outcome? The restraint was removed three hours later. The patient slept peacefully through the rest of the night. The nurse felt safe and comfortable during the time needed for her to assess the client's self-asserted change of condition. Her ability to understand both sides of the problem helped her to propose a solution that restored control to her client while maintaining necessary safety standards.

The second client has right-sided hemiparesis but refused assistance. He would lurch his way down the hall of his mobile home to the bathroom. His wife preferred that he stay in his room and use the urinal. She constantly admonished, "You'll fall, you'll fall." The nurse encouraged the wife not to discount her own needs and feelings but suggested that she change her phrasing to positive terms in order to avoid giving unintended indirect negative suggestions (11). For example, she could say, "I'm afraid when you go to the bathroom without my help. I want you to walk safely and continue to be as strong as you can be. I know how important being independent is to you. How can I help you get to the bathroom without worrying and also let you do it yourself?" He made the suggestion that solved the problem: he was willing to wear a heavy belt that she could hold onto without feeling that he was "leaning" on her.

Of course, any number of alternative solutions might have been tried in this situation. It is possible that after a reasonably full sharing of perspectives, the wife might have chosen not to worry so much, and the husband would have continued his practice of independent action. Our point is that there *are no final, fixed, and standardized ways for dealing with specific nursing care problems.* Inviting all possible client control has incredible power for mutual personal growth and an incremental assumption of ability to dialog with significant others in affiliated-individuation.

The promotion of client control, described in many ways in this section, is a major challenge to the nurse practitioner. She will have less difficulty meeting this challenge as she learns how to *model* and *role-model* her client's world. As indicated previously Table 11-6 provides additional ideas for promoting control.

PROMOTING STRENGTHS

The identification and promotion of an individual's strengths has a long history in nursing. While nurses have aimed to detect and support strengths (upon which a person may build and improve the state of health), medicine's aim has been to find and solve problems. The two complement each other very well.

When stressors mount, persons often lose sight of the strengths and capabilities they have in terms of who they are and their life exeriences. They invariably benefit when an alert nurse raises their awareness of their positive qualities and abilities. Many people deny that they have any strengths. Frequently, they will give no answers at all when asked "What are your strengths?" On the other hand, they are usually able to cite a long list of weaknesses without prompting.

Since people are often not aware of their own uniqueness, we have found it helpful to label and describe their strengths as frequently as possible. Strengths can be biological (you can breathe so well), cognitive (you certainly are a clear thinker), affective (you have a nice sense of what makes you angry), behavioral (you are gentle), physical (you are strong; you have a nice nose), abstract (you really are a special person), and so forth. We caution the nurse to be wise about identifying strengths while developing a trusting relationship. One general rule of thumb is this: You can almost always safely and wisely identify biological strengths without raising red flags in your client's mind. (The only exception here would be clients who are experiencing secondary gains from illness.) Many people who can't find much to value about themselves are suspicious if the nurse lists too many strengths. We have found that some people are able to incorporate only one new strength at a time; more than that seems to raise anxiety in them.

There are many subtle ways to identify and promote strengths. For example, when doing a physical examination you can describe your client's health status and strengths to him or her. As you assess a system, you can specify how strong the respirations are, how regular the heart beats are, and so forth. This technique is often overlooked by nurses, although many of them have had the experience of hearing "Um, UM, *UM!*" as the doctor or nurse listens to, palpates, or inspects our bodies. We always assume that this "Um, UM, *UM!*" means bad news. How reassuring it is to learn, instead, that it means we are healthy human beings.

We teach persons to identify and capitalize on as many positive and pleasurable feelings as they can, even when they are hospitalized. We sometimes describe the hypothalamic-pituitary-cortical effects on body chemistry and the immune system in particular, to help them understand how good feelings promote healing, help prevent disorder, and enhance existing states of health. We thereby affirm their power to help themselves through practicing these principles of self-care. They become fascinated learning about their own powerful internal tranquilizers, the endorphins. Some are interested in imagery and relaxation techniques (12). All of these "teachings" emerge from our active listening and in relation to the person's expressed wants and needs. All help specify strengths already in operation.

Sometimes we have had to search to find a strength to comment on (13). It has often been necessary to construct a base line in some creatively measurable way so as to be able to detect even the smallest change over time in feelings, structure, or function. For example, we can teach people to identify the severity of their discomforts, such as pain, nausea, itching, sleeplessness, sadness, by having them give these symptoms ratings on numerical scales, such as one to ten (worst possible). This makes it possible for them to rate and observe their own changes, thus becoming more aware of small improvements over shorter periods of time. It provides greater precision than such statements as "I think it's better, but I'm not sure." Such a quantified, measurable self-report can have a powerful effect because of the mind–body relationship.

We teach patients to be aware of their physiological and psychological discomforts, to think about and discover how they can directly or indirectly control these feelings. Indeed, control is identified as seeking assistance when needed. Clients learn that they can reach out more directly for what they want and need; that they do not have to suffer in order to be accepted and cared for. This ability to help themselves becomes a new and powerful strength, which we heartily reinforce. We tell them that the most independent person is the person who knows what he or she wants, where to get it—and then gets it. Simultaneously, we assure them that humans want to be good, to do their best, and will naturally strive toward a loving, sharing relationship with others when they have had their own needs met.

We find different ways to promote strengths, depending on how the client has modeled her world. Consider the client who enjoyed having her new strengths placed in a box and wrapped as a gift. We had learned that she liked gifts—she was constantly giving them to others—so *modeling her world*, and then *role-modeling* a healthier world, was easy. We listed her strengths, one at a time, wrapped them as gifts, and gave them to her. She gradually took on her new strengths and used them.

Techniques for promoting strengths are similar to those of identifying existing strengths but are more proactive. You, as a nurse, *role-model* for your client what his or her world can be like. For example, if your client seems generally to lack interpersonal closeness but you note that the client can be close to an animal or a pet (or even enjoy a plant), you can comment on the positive aspects of his or her relationship with the animal. Later you can comment on the behavior, identifying it as a strength. You would then observe any possible human exchange that might be linked to these associations and reinforce it. In this manner of linking and chaining behaviors, you can help your client gradually generalize positive behavior and gain control over negative behaviors by purposeful action. Ultimately, the client will improve the self-image and change his or her behavior with humans. Below is an example:

> We knew a client who would come into the nurse's office for weekly visits and rant and rave for the full hour about how tough and mean he was. He would tell his family what to do and what not to do; he "smacked" his kids for being "mouthy"; he nearly killed two men in a fight, and so on. His voice would get so loud he could be heard in the hall. His nurse listened patiently for two weeks to how "awful" he could be. At the beginning and end of each session she told him how nice it was to see him and gently patted him on the back as he prepared to leave the office. He arrived for his session on the third week, took his usual seat, and began his triade. After about 15 minutes of loud exclaiming, wild gesturing, and making the usual statements, he knocked a hooked rug off the wall. He immediately retrieved it and carefully replaced it on its hook, apologizing for "getting carried away again." The nurse told him she understood that he had a lot of strong feelings that he wanted to express, and that in due time he would learn to express these so that he felt he had control over his feelings rather than being controlled by them. She then added that she noticed how gentle he had been with the hooked rug, and how much she admired that gentleness. She immediately changed the subject, commenting that all humans have feelings, all people want to be the best they can be, and all people have needs. Sometimes these things get all mixed up and we only need someone to help us sort them out. When that happens, good things happen to us. She then commented that it was time for him to go, and that she would look forward to his return the next week.
>
> The following week he returned, commented that things had gone fairly well at his organizational meeting for a change, and he was feeling good. He had also lost five pounds (which was more than the goal he had set for himself the week before). The nurse commented that she was so pleased he had experienced a positive time and hoped that he had more enjoyable days ahead. She also commented that she knew there would be some

bad times—life was like that—but gentle people also had good times and good feelings. He looked her straight in the eye and responded that he wasn't a gentle person, whereupon she laughed and commented that he couldn't fool her; she had seen his gentleness the week before. Underneath, he was probably a lovely flower waiting to come out. Embarrassed, he laughed and commented, "I don't think so. But who knows?" While he sometimes would become loud and express his anger toward individuals in later sessions, he also became a more gentle person.

Perhaps more daringly we have made it a habit to identify the strengths we see in people, even when they are experiencing severe physical stressors such as dyspnea, postoperative pain, and so forth. We have been pleased that as we point out small advances, an ascending cycle of continued improvement occurs. We think that people's focusing on their discomforts blinds them to any real, although small, signs of health in themselves. Since their minds entertain only the "worst possible" outcomes, fight-flight reactions quickly follow. All these combine to make their contribution to a continuous, descending spiral. They snuff out the little biophysical gains before the latter have had time to consolidate.

For similar reasons, we measure wounds and describe them when our clients cannot see them. At all times we seek to encourage people to be true participant–executors in their own care. One really important—and often overlooked—strength is people's awareness of themselves, their reactions and responses and, if they are older, the intuition and wisdom developed over years of self-scrutiny. People often express their insights as truisms. These insights often relate to commonalities of human experience and many have recently been supported by research. When we cite studies that support the person's own lifelong observations, we help meet self-esteem needs through affirming these strengths. We continually work toward phrasing our comments and recommendations to clients as positively as possible in order to avoid any possible adverse effects from inadvertent indirect suggestions. We recall the following example:

A man collapsed in church, was carried out, and given mouth-to-mouth resuscitation in the narthex. Pale and visibly shaken after the experience, he staunchly insisted that he was all right now. The physician at his side was heard to say, "You'll have to go to the hospital for a check-up. This could be very dangerous." The nurse quickly added, "You're important enough that if, indeed, you're all right, you'll want to reassure yourself of that." The nurse's approach also takes into account a person's need to digest possible "bad news" at his or her own rate and timing. (The man went home with a "clean slate" after three days in the hospital for observation and multiple tests.)

Our opportunities to look for, comment on, compliment, describe, reinforce, commend, and raise consciousness levels regarding strengths is an exciting adventure as well as a powerful, deliberate means whereby self-care is promoted. We encourage you not to discount the smallest one. When you are not yet sure if an observation falls into the category of a "strength," resort to a simple description of what you see or hear or palpate. Begin with "I am aware that . . ." and you'll always be giving your client the benefit of the doubt while telling only the truth. Additional ideas for promoting strengths can be found in Table 11-7.

TABLE 11-7 Promoting Strengths at Every Level
of Maslow's Hierarchy

The following are representative examples of interventions designed to meet basic needs. Adapt them creatively to match your client's model of the world.

General Guidelines

1. Frequently "mirror" strengths and "normal" observations with:
   "I am aware that . . .
   "Are you aware that . . .
   "I note that . . .
   "I want you to notice . . .
   "Did you hear yourself . . .
   "What do *you* see . . .
   "May I share with you what I saw (my perception, my experience of you, what I heard, etc.) . . ."
2. Focus the client's existing sensory abilities upon natural beauties and common wonders, for example, the hovering of a hummingbird, exquisite detail of a flower, flight of a bird, shining stars, rhythm of ocean waves, warmth of sun, baby's smile, toddler's

TABLE 11-7 (Cont.)

chuckle, babbling of brook, fall colors, peacefulness of falling snow, sound of wind and rain, crackling of leaves underfoot.

While Meeting Biophysical Needs

1. As you examine physical parts, make remarks similar to the following:

   "Your pulse is strong and regular."

   "Your skin is smooth, moisture-filled, and unbroken (free of bruises, bumps), and it shows an active blood circulation."

   "Your eyes are shiny."

   "Your lungs are clear."

   "I hear your breath sounds moving in and out easily, smoothly, and evenly."

   "You are controlling your breaths, sometimes faster, sometimes slower."

   "Your wound is healing. The new tissue is pink and clean."

2. When picking up meal trays, comment on the specific foods eaten and their nutritional value to the client: "How beneficial that protein will be to help you heal faster!"

3. Praise client's efforts to "listen to his body," understand his health care needs, and participate in self-care.

While Meeting Safety and Security Needs

1. Praise and verbally approve the client's efforts to help guard her own safety by questioning procedures, medications the client is receiving, physicians, hospital policies, and so forth.

3. Identify questions the client asks about his or her health as self-care strengths. "You are like others who are taking more and more responsibility today for helping themselves feel better (or prevent disease)."

3. Teach other components of contemporary role as active health care consumer.

4. Help client learn that we are each responsible for our own feelings and have the ability to control them.

5. Help client learn that while we cannot *control* the responses of others, we can change them through changing our own behaviors that we *can* control.

6. Help client learn that we can give ourselves physical feelings and pains just as we give ourselves emotional feelings in our chosen response to others' actions and life events. Help client ask himself or herself (gently!) what gains he or she gets from particular symptoms, such as abdominal pains, headaches, and so forth. Ask the

TABLE 11-7 (Cont.)

client, "What is the benefit to you of such feelings?" Follow with, "Can you achieve this benefit by means less costly to yourself (with less personal discomfort)?" "What would happen if you. . . ?"

While Meeting Love and Belonging Needs

1. Identify specific ways in which members of client's support system have shown their caring, concern, and ability to help.
2. Laugh, tease, joke with the client whenever appropriate. Share brief, humorous relevant anecdotes and/or cartoons for mutual enjoyment.
3. Encourage significant others to relate normally to client with touch, words, humor, honest information, sharing feelings, and continuing ordinary discipline.
4. Suggest that the client make a list of strengths and traits he or she values in significant others.
5. Remind client to reinforce behaviors he or she appreciates from his or her support system by verbal and written means.

While Meeting Esteem and Self-Esteem Needs

1. Compliment the logic and wisdom the client shows in putting ideas, information, and experiences together to draw valid conclusions about self.
2. Explain how knowing one's feelings is a strength and learning to verbalize them can improve interpersonal communication skills in all contacts (family, work, community).
3. Use the following when they apply: "Are you aware what skillful choices you are making." (Detail them.) "These are strengths that you can always build on." "Everyone has feelings like that sometimes. How will you use this very useful information to your advantage?"
4. Reinforce any Eriksonian strengths or virtues identified.

SETTING HEALTH-DIRECTED GOALS

Remember that individuals have an innate drive to be as healthy as they can. You can depend on that motivation to work for your client. Disruptions in continued growth occur at any stage of life or in any situation in which the individual's basic needs are not met. Whatever the individual's "presenting problem" is, it is the unmet needs that are the nurse's focus. When the nurse assists the client in meeting those basic needs, the client will grow healthier. (Often the particular "presenting problem" will disappear.) In this general sense, the nurse's and the client's goals are the same: both want the basic needs met.

In the context of concrete settings and specific nurse–client encounters, it may appear that client goals and nursing goals differ. What may be happening is that the nurse is misreading (has not fully *modeled*) her client's *world*, including understanding what needs are unmet. We again present a favorite and particularly instructive story of ours (first presented in Chapter 10) concerning a woman whose mother was in a rehabilitation unit after surgery for a benign brain tumor. Expectations were that the mother would get better "really fast." Instead, she took out her hearing aid, became incontinent, refused to feed herself, and was generally acting "just terrible." Long-distance telephone calls communicated the nurses' despair, as they asked the patient's daughter what they could do with her. Consultation with the daughter about our paradigm led to the suggestion that if the mother were to be cared for within the context of our paradigm, the nurse on the unit would need to determine her unmet basic needs and current adaptive potential. The daughter was directed to have the nurses ask her mother these questions: "What is the problem?" "What do you think you are able to do for yourself?" "What can we (nurses) do to help you feel and get better?" The mother's response was, "What I need is a sitter." Understandably, the nurses were upset, given their worries about muscle atrophy and rapid decompensation of the woman's self-care activities. The daughter, believing in our paradigm, encouraged the nurses to agree to her mother's request. In accord with other components of the paradigm, she requested that when the sitter was provided the nurses acknowledge the mother's conviction that the sitter was intended to be helpful and also ask her, "When do you think you'll be ready to give up a sitter?"

Three days later the mother felt safe enough to give up her sitter. Two and a half months later she was living in Florida in her own apartment, happy and active.

In this example, the nurses were led to an understanding and appreciation of the client's real, unmet needs. The mutually defined goal was to meet those needs. The intervention, then, was to accede to the client's view of how to do that. In other situations, after discussion with a nurse, a client may announce a goal but have plans for its achievement that are either vague or overly ambitious. For example, a client may truly desire to lose weight without having much of a notion about what eating habits produce that outcome. Or the client may announce the desire to lose 20 pounds in two days. In such situations, as we help clients achieve their own goals, we need to take care that the steps are small enough and truly achievable in order to avoid failure and its attendant negative feelings. The "success breeds success" formula cannot be improved upon. For this reason, we often help a person scale the initial phrasing of a goal into a more manageable first step. Genuine approval, commendation, and reinforcement are provided when the client takes that first step. The process is repeated for subsequent small steps toward the goal until the goal is reached (14).

Whether goals are long or short range, they simply cannot be set without maximum participation on the part of the person we help. In helping the client to lose weight we can give information about calories and foods. The client, however, decides to give up the second donut for breakfast, but not donuts altogether. The nurse discusses with the client important principles within her scientific knowledge base related to goal attainment. To stay with the issue of losing weight, she discusses relationships between weight and calories taken in and calories burned. To better assure that she *models* the client's world, she asks, "What are you able to do to achieve your goal?" and "What can I do to be of help?" The client is willing to modify the amount eaten but not what he or she eats. The client asks, "Is that OK?" One can infer that the client is asking for the nurse to help by affirming the legitimacy of the plan. Her support of the client's willingness to take action to improve his or her own health will assist the client to move in that direction.

It is important to remember that to be "healthier" is not the same as achieving optimum health. In our example, the outcome of the nurse–client interaction is a healthier state for the client: eating habits have improved. Yet both share the view that the client is not at an optimum weight. Often there are changes over time in what the client is willing to do or in what the client wants from his or her nurse. The interactive and interpersonal process is repeated innumerable times as the nurse nurtures her client.

The above paragraphs described goals that we seek in response to basic-need deficits. Clients and nurses also work on goals that are of a longer range. Many of these are related to optimum-level task resolution. Sometimes clients are working on the task of autonomy, sometimes industry, and so forth. It is useful for the nurse to be cognizant of these goals. Many times the task resolution creates a crisis for the client (15). Nurses can use interventions that will assist the client in understanding the difficulty and identifying acceptable alternatives.

When nurses who have *modeled* their client's *world* consider developmental task resolution, they are able to predict possible future task resolution. Table 11-8 provides additional ideas for goal setting. We are certain that you can add to them.

TABLE 11-8   Mutual Goal Setting

Setting small, achievable goals requires a similar process, regardless of the level to which the goals are attached. First we list one useful sequence of nurse actions and follow with examples of the kind of goals we are talking about that are related to each level of the hierarchy. The latter will be phrased from the client's perspective—the desired outcome of an effective goal-setting dialog between the nurse and the client.

General Guidelines

1. Gain client's perception of a change he or she desires. (You may give initial information to activate the client's desire and concern.)
2. Verbalize the importance of choosing goals and priorities that can and will be kept.
3. Invite client's expression of what client thinks he or she can and will do for himself or herself.
4. If necessary, help the client scale back overly-ambitious goals to smaller, assuredly manageable steps. (It usually is necessary.) Mutually set the target time and date.
5. Explore with client what might interfere with or stop client from achieving his or her goal.
6. Assist the client in dealing with potential barriers. Alter plans accordingly.
7. Extend yourself as help or support in any specific way the client describes that you can comfortably accept.
8. Reinforce achievement of the goal. Praise, commend, approve, affirm, summarize, and acknowledge with such expressions as the following:
   "I'm pleased. . . ."
   "I like the way. . . ."
   "I like your. . . ."
   "I'm impressed. That's *hard* and you *did* it. . . ."
   "I find that (very responsible, wise, delightful, comical, etc.)."

TABLE 11-8 (Cont.)

9. "Reframe" partial achievements: "Let's look at the glass as half full, not half empty." "That's an important piece of information for you (for us both.)" "We can *use* what we've learned from this experience." "Let's see how much we can build from here." "Let's not discount what you *did* do." "How do you think we can build from here?" "What further ideas do you have?" "Would you like more input from me?" "Would some suggestions help to trigger your thinking?"

When Meeting Biophysical Needs (phrased as client's objectives)

1. Breathe more easily during the next ten minutes by using pursed-lip breathing.
2. Sleep without *any* interruptions for two hours.
3. Take medications five out of seven days this week.
4. Walk one mile three times this week.
5. Eat more slowly; take a half-hour for each meal.
6. Increase daily walk by five feet each time (each day, etc.).
7. Keep a record of fun activities done in a week.
8. Alter an identified patterned behavior by trying *anything* that is different one out of three times throughout the week (or today).
9. Pick up the novel and read at least five minutes, every time I'm tempted to open the refrigerator door.

When Meeting Safety and Security Needs (phrased as client's objectives)

1. Ask people to repeat what I don't understand.
2. Speak out once in a meeting next week.
3. Take a friend with me when I go jogging at dusk.
4. Ask for clarification when I don't understand, at least once this week.
5. Tell friends I'm looking for a watchdog.
6. Tell the doctor I want a second opinion.

When Meeting Love and Belonging Needs (phrased as client's objectives)

1. Tell husband one thing I appreciate four days out of seven this week.
2. List the advantages and disadvantages of having a roommate.
3. Directly express my feeling of anger without condemning the other person by using "I . . ." statements.
4. Request father to visit tomorrow.
5. Verbalize, "I love you *and* I also need more time to myself." (Not *but*.)

TABLE 11-8 (Cont.)

6. Spend ten minutes together without the children two times this week.

When Meeting Esteem and Self-Esteem Needs (phrased as client's objectives)

1. List five personal strengths I find myself using this week.
2. By tonight make a list of things I like to do.
3. Inquire about handicraft classes at the "Y" tomorrow morning.
4. Get haircut with money set aside from first paycheck.
5. Tell people the name by which I prefer to be called.
6. Introduce myself within one minute of entering room.
7. Read one page of the newspaper before attending a party.
8. Make up a list of 30 simple, inexpensive pleasures by this Friday.

SUMMARY

Five general *aims* shape all our nursing interventions. These are: (1) build trust, (2) promote client's positive orientation, (3) promote client's control, (4) affirm and promote client's strengths, and (5) set mutual goals that are health directed.

If nurses design interventions according to the five general *aims*, their nursing actions will be both theory-based and fully individualized to the client's needs.

We try to engage at least one intervention that reflects each general *aim* during every client contact. This means we often implement all five *aims* at one time. A single intervention specifically aimed at meeting one basic-need deficit often concurrently addresses one or more other levels of Maslow's hierarchy. That is, an intervention that reflects the *aim* of building trust may also meet the *aim* of promoting control. Similarly, an intervention designed to promote a positive orientation may increase a sense of security *and* physical comfort.

As we work from within our theory and paradigm, a complex interweaving of *aims*, needs, and specific interventions occurs. What results? A client whose self-care is effectively nurtured at conscious and unconscious levels in all aspects of his or her being and a nurse who is free to be maximally creative within the specific guidelines of a comprehensive theory and paradigm.

NOTES

1. Meyer Friedman and Ray Rosenman, *Type A Behavior and Your Heart* (Greenwich, Conn.: Fawcett Crest Books, 1974).
2. R. J. W. Burrell, "The Possible Bearing of Curse Death and Other Factors in Bantu Culture on the Etiology of Myocardial Infarction," in *The Etiology of Myocardial Infarction*, ed. T. N. James and J. W. Keyes (Boston: Little, Brown, 1963), pp. 95–97.
3. Colin Murray Parkes, *Bereavement: Studies of Grief in Adult Life* (New York: International University Press, 1972).
4. Sidney Jourard, "Suicide: An Invitation to Die," *American Journal of Nursing* 70 (1970): 269–75.
　　——, *The Transparent Self* (New York: Van Nostrand, 1971).
　　——, *Healthy Personality: An Approach from the Humanistic Viewpoint* (New York: Van Nostrand, 1974).
5. Take a baby learning to walk as an example. Anyone who has had the delight of watching can remember those first few steps. There is excitement, expectation, and fear on the baby's face as the baby takes that first big step. It's safe on the floor, but your knees get sore; you can't see very well; everything has a perpendicular perspective for you. On the other hand, if you walk, it's a long way down when you fall, but the world looks different up there. It's closer to your eye level; you have a horizontal perspective; and it's very exciting. Little does the baby "know" that he or she probably won't really get hurt if he or she falls, since from the baby's personal perspective it *does* hurt. While some babies probably learn to walk without reinforcement from their loved ones, most gain courage by having someone face them whose voice and smile is full of invitation and encouragement or by having someone to hang onto while trying this new, exciting step in life.
6. Clarice Kestenbaum, "The Origins of Affect—Normal and Pathological," *Journal of the American Academy of Psychoanalysis* 8 (1980): 497–519.
7. We use the client/patient term purposefully. The nurse caring for this individual treated her primarily as a patient. It was only when she was desperate that she resorted to asking the girl what *she* thought would help her! At this point, the nurse treated her as a client, but lacking a theory base, she didn't fully understand the importance of her own actions. As a result, she vacillated between treating people as patients and treating them as clients.

8. John Grinder and Richard Bandler, *The Structure of Magic II* (Palo Alto, Calif.: Science and Behavior Books, 1976).

9. Dorothy Babcock, "Transactional Analysis: An Introduction to some Basic Concepts of TA and its Usefulness to Nurses," *American Journal of Nursing* 15 (1976): 1153–55.

10. Stephen Karpman, "Fairy Tales and Script Drama Analysis," *Transactional Analysis Bulletin* 7 (1968): 39–43.

11. The expression "I'm afraid you'll fall" is related to the expression "Don't think about falling," in which the person cannot *not* think about the prohibited idea because of the admonition itself. It has been introduced to the person's conscious (and unconscious) mind by the well-intentioned speaker. To understand the usefulness of positive phrasing in our culture, consider the child learning to ride a bike whose father calls out, "Don't fall!" as compared to "Keep pedaling!" Similarly, the person who hears a warning that if he can't void, he'll be catheterized may be disadvantaged over one who is told, "As you relax more and more, you'll find your water flowing freely."

12. Patricia Flynn's, *Holistic Health: The Art and Science of Care* (Bowie, Md.: Brady, 1981), provides several techniques that might be helpful. Other resources include K. E. Claus and J. T. Bailey's *Living with Stress and Promoting Well-Being* (St. Louis: C. V. Mosby Co., 1980) and Gary Cooper's *The Stress Check: Coping with the Stress of Life and Work* (Englewood Cliffs, N.J.: Prentice-Hall, Spectrum Books, 1981).

13. Extreme situations, as when helping the suicidal and self-destructive person, provide a challenge to identify strengths. Yet it is possible to tell an unsuccessful overdoser that "some part of you is very strong and wants very much to survive and find a better way." One client who was berating herself for her inability to stop antagonizing her husband by automatically asking him, "*Why* do you *always. . .?*" learned that a strength lay in starting to realize what she had done *immediately* afterward.

14. Susan Steckel, *Patient Contracting* (Englewood Cliffs, N.J.: Prentice-Hall, Appleton-Century-Crofts, 1982). This is a detailed step by step guide that is especially helpful to nurses.

15. A classic reference for dealing with crises is D. Aguilera and J. Messiah's *Crisis Intervention: Theory and Methodology* (St. Louis: C. V. Mosby, 1982). Their sections on situational and maturational crises, pp. 73–177, are especially pertinent to this text.

12

What Do You Need to Practice Nursing?

OVERVIEW

In preceding chapters we presented our perspectives on why you need to think about your philosophy of nursing and learn to label and be articulate about your practice. We also presented our theory and paradigm for nursing practice. We now focus on what you will need to consider if you are to implement the modeling and role-modeling paradigm. These are:

1. Have confidence in nursing.
2. Establish a belief system.
3. Promote adherence.
4. Develop a language.
5. Give and get collegial support.
6. Be willing to take risks.
7. Believe in yourself.

Although we will address each of these independently of the others, the discussion throughout will demonstrate their overlap.

HAVE CONFIDENCE IN NURSING

We believe that before you can adopt this theory and paradigm for your nursing practice, you will need to be very clear in your own mind about the difference between nursing and other health professions. You will also need to sincerely believe that nursing is a profession that is vital for human welfare. This means that nursing is a unique and special profession and that practitioners of nursing are special and unique beings. Accepting that nursing has a separate and distinct contribution to make to health care may be a problem for some of you. We suffer from a long socialization process that reinforces the subservient role and the dependent functions of the nurse. For some, it is difficult to undo those attitudes, feelings, and thoughts.

We are not talking about the attitudes, feelings, and thoughts of our colleagues or consumers; we are talking about *your* attitudes, feelings, and thoughts. Some of these may be so well ingrained that you will have trouble seeing them as a source of difficulty. Some of you will choose not to see. That is certainly your choice. Nevertheless, before you dare to risk some of the ideas presented in this paradigm, you will need to see clearly what you are aiming for, and why.

Nursing is a profession that nurtures people. This means that your role as a nurse will be to promote the development of your client. Society has sent out double messages about this role since the beginning of our country. People are supposed to be big and strong, tough and independent (1). Societal contributions are valued in terms of what individuals are able to do for themselves and the changes they carve out in the material environment around them. Functions that support and maintain another's ability to act are hidden and therefore not valued. Furthermore, being independent has meant that individuals do not even need nurturance. Young children and the sick are seen as exceptions. Thus, the people (traditionally females) who fill nurturing roles are not valued since their presence symbolizes a feared state. It is as if nurturing roles are a "necessary evil." Someone must take care of the family, the children, and the sick, but these roles are not essential for the survival and progress of society.

Historically, women were encouraged to become professionals when it was determined that such entry into the world outside the home would benefit society. Generally, these "benefits" included cheaper labor, labor that would do the work at hand and not complain or become restless, labor that could be told how to do their work and when to do it. There have been few (if any) times that society has openly stated that the tasks delegated to women were essential or extremely important to human welfare. Although women were "permitted" to teach because they were natural nurturers of children and their minds, the main driving force for permitting entry was the fact that women could be hired more cheaply than men, and men were getting tired of such menial work and its low status.

The major professions filled by women are elementary education, nursing, and social work. All three professions focus on facilitating individuals in their own personal development; all three have traditionally been low-status positions. Perhaps the difficulty lies in the fact that the role of such professionals is to *facilitate*, not to *do*. We, however, urge you to acknowledge fully that no one acts without support. The ability to facilitate another's development is as creative an endeavor as perceived independent action. It too requires a profound understanding of how the world works. These services are absolutely necessary for the survival of society; therefore, individuals providing such services are vitally important.

If you are to practice a paradigm that clearly distinguishes nursing from other professions, then you must think through whether or not you really and truly believe that nursing is a service or function that is essential, not just useful, for the well-being of society. It is only after you have made this decision that you will have the fortitude to continuously explain to your colleagues what you think and what you believe about your profession.

ESTABLISH A BELIEF SYSTEM

We have urged you to think about your philosophy of nursing. We feel so strongly about this that we have separated it out as an issue to address in this section. When we talk about a philosophy and a belief system, we don't simply mean sitting around with your colleagues and discussing what nursing is all about, although that is really where such a process usually begins. Instead, we mean an in-depth searching in your heart, mind, and soul of what you really believe. Until you do this, you might have difficulty standing by your philosophy when things seem to go wrong. For example, when you are under pressure to make a decision and your client's goals differ from those of the doctor, you might fall back on old habits rather than make judgments based on your philosophy. Firm convictions go a long way in assisting you to practice consistently and to justify your interventions clearly.

As you work on this task, you will want to remember that you are human and that you will probably change some of your beliefs over time. Perhaps you won't change the essence of your philosophy, but you may change the way you operationalize it. That should be expected, applauded, and rewarded, since humans do change and grow over time. The point is this: we have repeatedly said that it is essential that we accept our clients where they are at any point in time. We are saying to you that the same holds true for you as a professional. You must give yourself room to grow, to think, to be. Without such permission you will experience an incongruence between your current thoughts and those of five years ago, as well as those of five years from now. To hold different views now does not mean you devalue yourself for the views you held five years ago. Those changes directly reflect that you, like all other humans, have an innate need to know, to grow, and to develop. Rejoice in your development and in what lies ahead.

PROMOTE ADHERENCE

A common concern in the health care literature today is how to promote patient compliance. Many health risks have been identified, as well as the relationship among these risk factors and illness states. We as health care providers have become acutely aware of these relationships and have sought ways to effect compliance with health care plans. We nurses have talked considerably about the role of the nurse as a "patient educator." We do all of these things because we sincerely and honestly care about our consumers, just as our colleagues in other professions honestly and sincerely care about their consumers. Nevertheless, with all of our caring, all of our knowledge, and all of our concern, people still indulge in high-risk behaviors. We still eat too much, exercise too little, smoke, drink, and so forth. Some of us do these things and stay healthy; some don't.

The problem is very simple. Our consumers don't really believe in our "high-risk factors" *for their world*, not the way they want that world modeled. Until they do, they will probably not change their lifestyles and attitudes, and they most certainly won't change just because we want them to. Finally, who knows what is really most effective (effective, remember; not right or wrong) for the welfare of the client? While there is indisputable evidence that smoking is bad for us, there is also evidence that too many changes undertaken too quickly can also be associated with illness. Nurse investigators have shown that they were unable to influence post-heart-attack patients who were in a state of *impoverishment* to quit smoking, but they were able to influence such changes in clients in the states of *equilibrium* and *arousal* (2). We believe that these *impoverished* persons did not have the necessary energy to cope with the stress produced by the efforts to quit smoking. Therefore, they continued their maladaptive patterns—at their own cost. If these individuals had been in a system where they would have been discounted or criticized or even threatened with rejection if they continued to smoke, they would have been stressed even further by the very intervention that was intended to make them better.

When terminally ill people were interviewed to determine what they thought had caused their illness, what they thought that they could do about it, and what their expectations of the outcome would be, *their model* was very different from the view espoused by their nurse (3). Who is correct?

We have made the point throughout the book that our paradigm requires that we *model* and *role-model* our *client's world*. We are now stating that implicit in this statement is the fact that compliance, in the true sense of the word, is incompatible with our philosophy. *Compliance* comes from the word comply, which is defined in the dictionary as, "to act in accordance with a request, an order, rule, etc.; to be formally polite." We do not believe that practicing our nursing paradigm would lead you to expect compliance as an appropriate behavior for your client. Compliance connotes that you are working with a patient, not with a client.

We encourage you to promote adherence. *Adhere* means "to stick fast, to stay attached, to firmly support; adherence is the act of sticking fast." We believe that your clients often need support and reinforcement to "stick fast" to a health care plan, even one that they have developed. They need you as a facilitator to assist them in the process. This need for support in order to adhere is evident in society. There are Weight Watchers, Alcoholics Anonymous, and other such groups that have been formed for this very reason. We therefore encourage nurses, who are naturals for this role, to assist individuals in adhering to those tasks they deem important to achieve their life goals.

DEVELOP A LANGUAGE

We need to learn how to talk to one another in a language that is understood by our colleagues in nursing. We would feel delighted if other professionals also understood us, but most important is that we understand one another. We probably already have a common, cursory language that we can use among ourselves and among our other colleagues, but it is superficial and nonspecific. For example, when we use the word role-model, many of you before reading this book might have thought that we meant setting a good example. We assume that you are clear in your mind by now that we do not mean simply setting a good example. But it is only after elaboration that you would know that we mean something other than the usual definition of the word. We need to learn to elaborate and consolidate our language. This is not to say that all nurses will speak the same language, either. Take, for example, psychology. In this field several languages are spoken, and each branch of psychology has its own language. Nevertheless, all psychologists have an understanding of the language used in each branch of psychology. These professionals started with the common agreement that their purpose for being had a specific focus, and then they proceeded to study the phenomena within that focus, to label and articulate those phenomena. Now they have a common language within their specialties.

We nurses need a common language. If we are to practice nursing from a theory base, utilizing a specific paradigm, we must be able to speak the language.

GIVE AND GET COLLEGIAL SUPPORT

Although this category in some respects overlaps other categories, it warrants special attention. We have been socialized to respect our colleagues, the doctors. We are learning that our consumers also warrant our respect and, in fact, deserve our focus of attention. We have, however, been very negligent in learning how to give and get support from our own nursing colleagues. It seems to us that nurses should not seek their support from their medical colleagues, but instead should seek it from their nursing colleagues. Although we will always want to seek emotional support from a variety of sources, and although we will always enjoy having others tell us that we are good nurses, we would benefit in our thrust for autonomy if we turned to our professional colleagues and our consumers for validation and support.

To say this another way, nurses will have difficulty practicing in an autonomous, collegial manner (as we depicted in Figure 1-1), unless their nursing colleagues support them in such roles. We have had several experiences in which we have tried to practice autonomous nursing within a system in which our nurse colleagues have either overtly or covertly sabotaged our interventions. Sometimes these nurses were practicing from a "medical model," and sometimes they were not. Nevertheless, such sabotaging interferes with the advancement of our profession.

We urge you to consider ways in which we nurses can learn to both give and get support from our own professional colleagues. With such support, we will be able to practice a nursing paradigm without difficulty.

BE WILLING TO TAKE RISKS

The nurse who courageously thinks through her beliefs, develops a philosophy, and then decides that her philosophy is compatible with our paradigm and is operationalized within our paradigm will probably want to implement it. This nurse will find herself not only somewhat excited but also a little anxious. What if her nursing diagnoses or her interventions are thought of as ridiculous, or not important? What does she do then? Worse yet, what if her nursing interventions are in disagreement with the doctors? (Remember the dog under the sheets?) Sometimes, her interventions might even be considered "spooky." What will this nurse do?

The first thing she will do is to go back and think about her philosophy, about her definition of nursing and the paradigm or theory base from which she is working. Upon consideration, if her interventions are theoretically sound, she will proceed. If necessary, she will seek reinforcement from her colleagues (nurses), and, of course, she will confirm her plan with her client. She will attempt to explain, describe, and articulate to her medical colleagues what she is doing and why she is doing it. Hopefully, such measures will resolve the problem, but sometimes they won't. At this time, the risk-taker nurse will have to decide whether she can get her client's needs met in a way that is compatible with others' goals and expectations or stick to her guns. Sometimes she will be able to alter her intervention slightly, so that it is acceptable (and she will know when it is acceptable by *modeling* the doctors' world) and sometimes she will have to hang in there and continue with her planned intervention. Each nurse will have to make these decisions for herself. The point is this: being different and standing up for what you believe and think is risky. Sometimes you may find yourself isolated and alone.

When this happens, you will be able to get your support from knowing that you and your client believe in what is right for the client as a unique person. *Who else really counts anyway?*

We remember the "good old days" when parents weren't allowed in their children's hospital rooms except during visiting hours, and some were discouraged from visiting even then. Some nurses who were client-oriented (rather than doctor- or system-oriented) would break the rules, because they knew how much better their small clients did when mommy or daddy was with them. Those nurses were risk takers, and they paved the way for the rest of us. They were also keenly aware of the importance of *modeling* the *child's world* if they were to be help the child most effectively. Since then, theorists such as Bowlby have studied the effects of such desertions on children and have found that these risk-taking nurses intuitively knew what needed to be done. Today we talk about object relations theory, morbid grieving, loss, and so forth; today we have a language for these phenomena so that we can speak to one another and state specifically what our risk-taking nurses knew all along.

To practice this paradigm, you will have to be a risk taker to some extent, since there will always be those who simply won't understand what you have "seen" all along. But there can be recognition too for one's effectiveness. We've learned to enjoy our doctor friends who say that we practice wizardry or are spooky, or who say, "I don't know what you mean; just tell me what to do." Such mutually accepting relationships come slowly, but they are certainly worth the work and the risk.

BELIEF IN YOURSELF

Unless you really, truly, believe in yourself, all the preceding comments will be lost on you. You are an essential, valued human being who knows how to practice your profession expertly. Believe that, and you've got it made! Go stand in front of the mirror, pull your shoulders back, and say "I'm OK!" (4). You'll be surprised what that will do, if you believe in it. If you don't, then you need to step outside yourself, figure out what world you have modeled for yourself, and what you can do about it. You may want to talk this over with a friend, colleague, or professional. Or do whatever you feel is helpful. We believe in you; believe in yourself.

SUMMARY

Nursing fulfills an absolutely essential function in our society. Thus nurses are vitally important to the welfare of their fellow human beings. A nurse's role is to nurture development in others. To assume this role requires that you develop a philosophy of nursing that supports this valued function. To promote development means to accept persons, including yourself, for what they are now and to assist them to become what they want to be. If you can adopt this perspective, you will be able to truly help your clients, your colleagues, and yourself. Learn to believe in yourself, your potential, your inherent value, and accept the value and potential in others and you're on your way to a lifetime of enjoyment within your profession.

NOTES

1. These messages, called Drivers by transactional analysts, are described by Taibi Kahler and Hedges Capers, "The Miniscript," *Transactional Analysis Bulletin* 4 (January, 1974), pp. 26–42.

2. Janis Boudreau Campbell and Nancy Leipold, "An Experimental Test of a Nurse-Designed Stop Smoking Program," research funded by W. W. Kellogg Foundation, paper presented at R. Faye McCain Research Symposium, University of Michigan, November 1979.

3. Barbara Kennison, "Nurses and Patients: The Clinical Reality of Sickness," a preliminary report of findings presented to the Ninth Annual Research Symposium, University of Michigan Graduate Programs in Nursing, April 29, 1982.

4. Thomas A. Harris, *I'm OK—You're OK: A Practical Guide to Transactional Analysis* (New York: Harper & Row, 1967).

IV

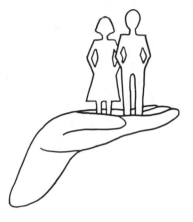

COMMON QUESTIONS

This final section contains a few of the questions commonly asked about our theory and paradigm. We present these here in hopes that they will further assist you in using our ideas. We encourage you to send us additional questions, comments, and ideas. We will respond as quickly as possible.

Q1: You build a good argument for psychosocial nursing. However, as a hospital nurse, I must be concerned about the safety of the patient's physical state. What do you say about that?

We welcome the opportunity to say again as clearly as we can that we are not talking about psychosocial nursing, or medical–surgical nursing, or any other kind of partial nursing. We do not believe that nursing is accurately described in partial terms that derive from a medical treatment model. In our opinion, nursing always includes the whole person in all respects. So, of course, we are concerned with you that a person's safety in all respects—physical state included—would be considered and attended to.

We regret that many of us have been burdened during socialization into the profession with a false conviction that we are personally and almost exclusively responsible to be on constant alert as if the client's safety rested primarily upon our ability to be aware of all dangers, to invariably make timely observations and intercept dangers of all kinds in an almost magical manner. Some of us even got the idea that we must so master a knowledge of medicine along with our other studies that we could monitor the physician's treatment plan in order to correct any omissions or incompatibilities committed by a distracted, fatigued, or careless medical practitioner. That is a human impossibility and we think nurses ought not to continue to

believe themselves superhumanly constituted or educationally prepared to take on such unrealistic responsibilities.

We think the truth is that most clients can be relied upon to
alert the nurse to impending difficulties *if* they feel the nurse's concern and support and know that their input to her—even "false
alarms"—will be heard carefully and taken seriously, without discounting of any kind. In this way, responsibility for safety rests
most heavily on clients and secondarily on the nurse who supports
the clients in their efforts to take the safest and best possible care
of themselves.

Take the use of cardiac drugs, for example. Years ago, when
drugs were limited in number and nature, nurses could learn a
special safety rule for administering a particularly potent one, such
as digitalis, and thought themselves able to take full responsibility
for observing its specific effects on a particular patient. Laying
aside the issue of when and how the client is going to learn the
medical facts he or she will need to use in daily self-care at home,
today we dare not pretend an unrealistic ability to personally and
independently monitor all possible interactions and dangers that
could result from the drugs we give. We, and the clients we serve,
no longer deal with an occasional cardiotonic, but with antiar-
rhythmics of varying mechanisms, antihypertensives, electrolyte
replacements, tranquilizers, chemotherapeutics, antibiotics, contra-
ceptives, muscle relaxants, narcotics, and so forth—all with potentially drastic single and interactive effects. Even the old standby
aspirin, formerly considered so safe, has synergistic effects that
present unexpected dangers to particular clients.

Of course, we nurses will do our homework in normal physiology, pharmacology, physical assessment, principles of physics,
and other subjects relating to the biophysical care of our clients.
Whenever we do not have answers to important questions, we will
be quick to consult our resources, both written and human. But
we cannot be walking encyclopedias. As we teach clients to accept
responsibility for observing and safeguarding themselves, we will
be scaling our own involvement in safety issues to manageable
realities.

Whenever a client is in known and certain jeopardy and unable
to act in his or her own behalf, and whenever that jeopardy can be
stemmed by the action of a nurse, such action must be taken by her.
The key words, however, are *known* and *certain* and *unable*. In
gray areas, when a nurse may not be sure, but still feels uncomfort-

able, she may share her discomfort with involved parties, client(s), physician(s), other nurses on the team—and act upon it—with clear explanations for the reasons behind her actions, including honest expressions of *whose* particular needs she may be meeting.

It is still important to tell the suicidal or aggressively destructive client, "I will not let you hurt yourself," or "We will not allow you to hurt others here." Items or equipment that might be used to injure self or others will still need to be removed from the scene. When physical restraints are needed to increase the peace of mind of either client(s) or care giver(s) or both, that must be faced honestly.

Of course, physical safety must be taken seriously. If the client really does not *know* that 17 candy bars consumed at one time can adversely affect the blood sugar, that information needs to be shared, respectfully, and caringly. If the client is unwilling to ambulate or cough and deep breathe after surgery, we need to express our concern directly without threat of withdrawal or abandonment. When we cannot think of more creative and effective ways to motivate the client within the client's model (when we feel stumped), we will use that feeling to take ourselves to a nursing colleague for our own support and consultation. But we say again, it is *not* the nurse's role to define for the client what the client will need nursing assistance for. That is for the client to say and the client will usually initiate specific nursing interventions and mutual small goal-setting through the sharing that occurs because the client feels trust in the nurse and feels trusted by her.

Emergency room nurses face special temptations to divide their nursing care into compartments of biophysical and psychosocial care. We do not deny the sometimes prior importance of acting instantly to alleviate severely compromised biophysical function, through supplying a critical substance or procedure that can mean the difference between sudden death and life. But when a physician is present in such cases, it is the physician's primary concern to deal intensively with those biophysical needs. During the time the nurse assists with any technical care (and as she becomes ever more efficient with specific equipment and medications she uses repeatedly in her unit), we think she can give crucially significant nursing to clients by deliberately, and purposefully attending to the *never-abrogated* interfacing of unmet biophysical needs with those of safety and security, love and belonging and, yes, even esteem and self-esteem. If the nurse does not give attention to the client's fears while he or she is receiving rapid-fire, frighteningly invasive, and painful care, the most efficient and smoothly executed technique may not produce its intended benefit. The challenge to emergency room nurses is to keep the holistic nature of the client and his or her possible unmet needs clearly in mind and hand, and to act deliberately to convey simultaneously a sense of security, affection, and esteem that may be the only way to invite a petrified client to "make it through" his or her personal ordeal.

We remember the burn physician who wrote in a nursing publication that the health team can pay attention to psychosocial needs after physical ones have been met. That is an understandable viewpoint on the part of a physician. It is not, however, to be taken as a mandate for nurses who ought to know better, and who *can* pull it all together by developing, when they choose, an ever-increasing expertise in the exercise of holistic care. It does not take a "sit-down" assessment of client needs to engage on-the-spot interventions according to the five general *aims*. Strengths can be affirmed even when clients are unconscious, or badly burned, or emerging from the coma of an overdose ("A part of you really wants to live and learn to do things differently"). Control can be given even to two-year-olds who sometimes know better than adults that *both* daddy and mommy are needed while *this* wound is being sutured.

Q2: You keep referring to being concerned with what concerns the client. I want to know how I can reconcile focusing attention on the client's concern if he or she is denying a very real and important problem, such as a bad heart, obesity, a destructive smoking habit, or a delusional system. How can I live with my own conscience if I don't point it out to the client and at least ask the client what he or she plans to do about it?

First of all, we remember that our job as nurses is to be perceived by the client as "on the client's side." We are naturally also on the side of the client's health—a state that does enjoy a certain consensual validation among health professionals. Also, because of our philosophy of nursing, we do indeed have values of our own. In our practices we have found it preeminently important to respect the client's own timing for acknowledging aspects of their health needs that they may not be ready to deal with at the time that they come for nursing care.

Practically speaking, most people already know what they need to "do something about." When we *say* it to them, we are often meeting our own needs to discharge our obligations to fellow professionals, who might charge us with being unaware or neglectful of issues they perceive must be handled by the client at some point in time. If we suggest to the client that he or she *ought* to be working on something, we become part of the stress under which the client already labors ineffectively.

The nature of nursing is to support the person, *where he or she currently is*, so that the person can reach the point of readiness and ability to follow recommendations from physicians and other professionals for changes he or she learns to know will promote health. It all depends on whether we are practicing nursing or medicine, or social work or psychotherapy. Given our theory of the relationship of human needs, object losses, and adaptive potential to growth and development, we will only add to the stressors people already experience if we are critically parental with them. As we showed in the example at the end of Chapter 8, clients will move forward toward health in a manner that promotes their interim safety and security *if* we support them with acceptance, information, and assistance according to their current coping states.

When the client presents what becomes a real problem to us by asking us to participate in some behavior that is ethically or morally repugnant to us, we do honestly acknowledge that such is a problem to us. We express it that way, owning it as our own problem and sharing our perspective sensitively with the client in the hope that we can negotiate a mutually acceptable compromise with the client.

In rare instances in which an irreconcilable conflict of values arises, we may have to withdraw from the relationship. Our hope is that this might be done in a spirit of mutual respect without creating or precipitating in the client a sense of having been abandoned for punitive reasons. The idea to convey is, "I cannot agree with what you have asked. I must therefore withdraw. I wish it were otherwise. I still care about you and what happens to you. I wish you well and hope you will find effective and constructive solutions to the concerns you are struggling with . . . and someone who may, in good conscience, be able to be a help to you."

Q3: As a staff nurse responsible for many patients concurrently, how can I possibly give the kind of individualized care I think you're advocating?

There seems to be an assumption here that individualized care necessarily takes more time to give than present common approaches. When we have acted to meet people's unmet needs by way of the five general *aims*, the ripple-out effect comes into play. As people's self-care actions are supported, they actually take less, not more, nursing time.

Let us set forth a number of related thoughts, observations, and principles deriving from our personal experience in busy wards. As you integrate these ideas, perhaps you will see your way clearer to at least *begin* practicing according to our paradigm and observe for yourselves the overall effect on your total unit's functioning.

1. Setting priorities is always in order and needed, regardless of the paradigm one practices.
2. People who are on the priority list for attention can often be helped to assume greater self-care responsibility.
3. Persons who feel their basic needs are being met by nurses rarely, if ever, complain about whether or not hotel-like functions are completed for them each day (daily changes of bed linens, delivery of fresh water on schedule, etc.). Since they feel infinitely more "cared about," they have fewer peripheral requests, complaints, or demands.
4. Basic needs can often be met in a very few actual minutes of care, assuming that a clear and purposive theory and paradigm are employed. If a substantial block of time *is* taken, it may in the long run preserve the nursing staff from even greater investments of time and energy extended over numerous future times. More strenuous efforts become necessary when complications occur that might otherwise have been avoided.
5. Persons with high self-care action potential can do many more things for themselves than we traditionally encourage, for example: keeping track of their own intake–output records, changing their own dressings, monitoring their own intravenous fluid flow rates, and even keeping their own charts and records. They are often personally benefited by helping with the simple and fully safe aspects of their own care, and in special instances, the care of their roommates (ward mates) as well.
6. Relatives and significant others can and often need to be incorporated into treatment and care regimes if their world is *modeled* and *role-modeled*. Heading off problems early will save much nursing time that would otherwise be used for patch-up, back-pedaling, and wheel-spinning operations to deal with full-blown "problem patients" and "problem relatives."
7. Well-cared for clients (a) heal faster, (b) learn self-care more

rapidly, (c) leave units earlier in better condition, prepared to continue self-care at home, and (d) return less often for complications and repeated hospitalizations.

8. Giving oneself permission to practice by the paradigm, with some clients at least, provides an opportunity for developing increasing skill and comfort in using it. In time, one's efforts may be expanded to include more clients. Learning is naturally and most comfortably a step-by-step process.

Q4: Can a person actually go back and complete a hitherto incomplete developmental task?

Yes, given two prerequisites: (a) an attachment figure who cares, accepts, understands, and who won't judge, react, or abandon and (b) the development of a trusting relationship (not merely a state of trust) with that attachment figure.

The appropriate attachment figure will have the strength and wisdom not to take any angry rejections from the client personally but to deal with the process occurring between nurse and client. The client may indeed test the consistent caring of the nurse in order to *prove* that the care giver cannot be "turned off" and to establish that the nurse will not reject despite the most provocative behavior. This is done to undo earlier messages from significant attachment figures who instructed, "Don't be you!" (or else I won't like you; or I'll leave you; or I'll stop taking care of you, and so forth).

Once the trusting relationship is firm, the client will risk looking at new options. With a decrease in tensions arising from the deletion of self-scolding and self-deprecating behaviors, the client will begin risking different behaviors and begin acting contrary to "old" internal messages such as *work hard, be perfect, please me, hurry up, be strong,* all of which are conditional acceptances (Chap. 12, note 1).

The client will begin "seeing" current realities without overlappings from "ancient" unresolved feelings. The client will become increasingly aware of his or her own feelings, accepting them without false guilt. The client will risk reaching out to do good things for himself or herself; to ask others for help needed at times; to offer to help others less compulsively and more appropriately; and to be able to alter his or her feelings through exchanging them for others via the deliberate use of cognitive skills.

As good things happen as an outcome of the exercise of an

increasing autonomy, the associated *strength* of self-control and *virtue* of will power will become more apparent. With the continuing support of the nurse, there can be a steady progressive movement through each successive unfinished task. This movement will be marked by the observable presence of the respective *strengths* and *virtues* identified by Erikson.

Q5: What guides can a young nurse follow in knowing when to collect a full data base and when not to? When can a nurse intervene without a full data base and when is it not all right?

Your questions assume at least two things: First, there is some objective standard for a full data base. Second, there are times when the *amount* of data permits interventions and times when it does not.

We submit that no one knows or ever will know what constitutes a full data base for nursing interventions. That will always depend on the individual client who may be unable or refusing to verbalize or otherwise reveal what would ordinarily (by other frameworks for care) be considered essential to design interventions. Nurses work with whatever is given them by the client who controls what is "full" or sufficient data. Let us ask a counterquestion. How much data on unmet basic needs is needed before action may be taken? The issue is whether or not sufficient *significant* data have been collected to plan interventions that produce effective outcomes. We remember that such outcomes are judged effective *by the client* who *perceives* the filling of an unmet basic need. Obtaining more data does not necessarily mean better interventions.

Your second question implies that there are not only specific amounts of data to be desired but also there are "right" and "wrong" times, as well as ways, to intervene in nursing—based in some way on the amount of data collected. We would suggest that helping in nursing is either effective or ineffective, not really "right" or "wrong." Remember too that nursing interventions *can* begin immediately. For example, our listening is an intervention that releases the client's stores of self-care knowledge, resources, and action. If our other interventions are ineffective, we will, by that very token, know that some additional data are needed. A client will probably not agree to a proposed plan to prevent bedsores if it is based on "insufficient" data.

The client, then, controls the amount of data given from which nursing interventions are designed. Ideally, the nurse imposes nothing on the client. If indeed she does, despite her best intention, this self-same "ineffective" behavior may be handled by starting over, this time listening, looking, and touching even more thoughtfully to elicit a clearer picture of the *client's own world*. We are, we remind ourselves, talking about nursing care, not about medical diagnosis and treatment.

These general comments aside, let us look briefly at the questions from the perspective of the client's *adaptive potential* (coping state). Very little data may be needed if clients can ask directly for what they want or need from nurses. This is true of many persons who are in *adaptive equilibrium*. If a person is *impoverished* or even out of contact with reality (as consensually validated), when will you know you have enough data to act? How will you get all you need? You will answer those questions by meeting your own needs along with the ones you associate with the client. You will need sufficient relevant data to *model* the *client's world* and simultaneously take into account your own basic needs, for example, to preserve your self-esteem as a safe or effective nurse. At times, particularly when persons are unconscious, the nurse uses her observations and available input from relatives to judge the sufficiency of the data for interventions that "take time" to plan. Fortunately, as the nurse follows the general aims of interventions, some on-the-spot interventions will meet individualized basic needs in a targeted way, whether or not the nurse ever learns objectively what those specific ways were. We think nurses must be allowed and encouraged to act on their theory base even if data are not "complete." Even the most comprehensive data base will have its areas of "objective" incompleteness.

We have found that when the client perceives the nurse has helped meet a currently expressed basic-need deficit, the client successfully reveals other needs in a sequence and timing that assures his or her interim safety while ultimately working toward holistic health.

Q6: How is it possible to view a 50-year-old as acting like a two-year-old? The person is an adult. Isn't the person supposed to be acting like one?

Well, of course, in some ways the person does, but in other ways not. We have sometimes explained the "incomplete task" in terms of a series of stacked boxes representing the tasks appropriate to a person's chronological age. It's as if the bottoms of several of the upper boxes have missing pieces through which the contents entering the top box filter down to a box whose bottom is more complete. Some storage is indeed possible but the capacities of the boxes are compromised so long as there are missing pieces. For those who find it difficult to understand basic needs and developmental tasks with this example, perhaps an analogy from the plant world using a living organism will help.

As a plant receives satisfaction of its basic needs for water, warmth, nutrients, sunlight, and protection from the elements through its attachment to the soil, it grows (meeting its potential) in a predictable fashion, sending out first a slender, and then a sturdier stalk, leaves, and later buds, flowers, and fruits. If a particular basic need is imperfectly met, say, for example, a part of the root system enters an unsuitable region, sustains damages, or meets other interference as with water supply, the portion of the above-ground plant that depends on that root section for its essential supplies, will show signs of deprivation. It may continue a kind of growth, but without optimum sturdiness, shape, and form, resistance to disease, and later, bud, blossom, and fruiting capacities. It may be able to draw some essential supplies from collateral areas and in the process may shortchange an adjacent segment from which it borrows. At some point the basic blockage of supplies of essential elements may be corrected (replanting may take place or irrigation, sunlight, and environmental conditions may improve) and invigoration may occur. The stalk may toughen up, become strengthened, and bear fruit, although it will probably always bear some mark of its earlier deprivation.

The plant is indeed always vulnerable to external stressors that are unrelated to its roots or early history in attachment to the earth. High winds, cold, scorching sun, drought, and human and animal predators may appear and exert their effect. The stronger the original plant, the more resources at its disposal for fending off or surviving the deleterious effects of these external stressors.

Simply stated, then, the 50-year-old who acts like a 2-year-old might be compared with the plant that showed evidence of deprivation secondary to unmet needs. Once these needs are consistently met, growth and development follow.

Q7: Do you distinguish between *modeling* and a person's *model* or perspective of his or her life/world?

Yes, the person's perspectives are very important and the most vital aspect of *modeling*. But in addition to these perspectives, we must consider our observations and whenever possible the perspectives of the family and other health care team members. These additional factors are indeed also a part of the *client's world* and therefore make their contributions to a full representation or model of it.

Finally, when one models, all data are analyzed using the theoretical formulations presented. Thus, diagnoses are derived from all the data gathered in the *modeling* phase.

Q8: What is the total range of self-care tasks that a person can do?

It all depends on the person's state of coping. If the individual is extremely *impoverished*, he or she might be fighting for life. At this time, the person might be able to do little more than such things as breathe, circulate blood, hear, feel, smell, or see. These strengths may be affirmed even as the nurse does many other physical care tasks for her client.

Persons in *arousal* can often do quite a bit for themselves if they receive support from nurses in the way of reminders of their strengths, past coping strategies, and current resources. Persons in *arousal* report themselves to be "tense-anxious." Their anxiety may be felt so acutely at the time that various existing skills and resources may be temporarily forgotten. A little reminding and encouragement for those existing strengths can go a long way. Many thereafter reach out effectively to arrange for whatever they want or need from others to stabilize themselves.

If persons are in *equilibrium*—and if their basic needs relating to all their subsystems are receiving care—they may go as far as to scrub their own deep abdominal wounds, catheterize themselves, feed themselves by tubes into the stomach or veins, mechanically suction their respiratory secretions, give themselves injections, decide dosage changes of medications they take, and so forth, according to the principles they have been taught.

In the future many more skills may be taught to people. Remember that the thermometer was once reserved for use by the physician alone. Today, with sufficient teaching and support, persons give themselves artificial kidney treatments at home.

The fact that treatments and procedures can indeed be done safely by anyone who is properly taught, even the client, helps to confirm that nursing does *not* consist of manual or technical expertise. As technically proficient nurses generously share that expertise, not only with clients, but also with colleagues who need to learn these skills, we are all freed to concentrate on making together the refined observations and evaluations of actions and intuitions critical to the development of that specialized body of nursing knowledge. This will include detailed mapping of the parameters of truly healthy structure and function. When we no longer equate skillful nursing with procedures per se, the ensuing increase of collegial respect and trust will help us welcome our differences and respective creative efforts. We will validate one another for providing effective *nursing* that supports the person's holistic self-care. That kind of nursing can never be minutely standardized or automatically and impersonally delivered.

Q9: **I am a primary care nurse in a health maintenance organization. I perform many routine physical examinations as part of my daily contacts with clients. I also prescribe medicines according to a preestablished protocol for minor ailments. Some nurse colleagues think that I am practicing "mini-medicine" or functioning as a physician's assistant. But I still think of myself as a nurse and think I am bringing nursing skills to my work.** *In the light of your ideas about self-care and the place of comprehensive examinations in the delivery of nursing care, would you agree with me or my critics?*

We think a consistent case might be made for the continuing performance of nursing in a setting such as you describe under several conditions. These involve keeping clearly in your mind the nursing focus, goal, and means of the care you provide. As you focus on a person and nurture that person's capacity to take better care of himself or herself, we think you might be able to use the "task" of physical examination to serve these ends.

What would happen if you briefly explained nursing's goal of facilitating self-care for growth and development, invited expression of any needs and concerns, and then did your physical examinations as a "helper alongside" of your client, continually looking for and taking advantage of opportunities to engage the five *aims*, sharing with the client—according to his or her readiness and willingness (need for and fear of knowledge)—the principles and rationale behind the observations you make and your decisions, *including the protocol you use in prescribing medicines?* Just openly sharing with the client that such a protocol exists and that *you will use it together* may correct any perception the client may hold that your expertise is "just like a doctor's." It also avoids reinforcing a common notion that health is something one entrusts to someone else for full care. Could a client thus be helped to understand that your goal is to enter a nurse-client relationship that will help the client take better care of himself or herself holistically? Will the client learn that this includes using standardly prescribed medications responsibly along with other measures that are all under his or her ultimate control?

Q10: Do doctors ever *model* and *role-model?*

We recall the story about the patient who was admitted to the hospital in an acute hypertensive crisis. The physician was deeply perplexed because the patient had been on medication and was doing very well. When asked if he had been taking his medication, the patient adamantly affirmed that he had indeed. Nevertheless, after he was hospitalized and the same medications were given by the staff, his blood pressure returned to normal.

One day as the doctor was leaving the room the patient asked when the doctor planned to flush out the poisons. The physician, intuitively realizing that this individual's model of the ongoing events differed from his, asked, "Poisons?" The patient then reported that everyone knew that hypertension medications were poison and needed to be "flushed out—otherwise bad things happened!" He went on to say that while at home he accomplished this by taking his pills for six months and then flushing his system for six months. Although the doctor and nurses had explained that he should stay on his medication continuously, it never occurred to him that his six months off was not taking his pills—it was merely taking good care of himself, within his *own model of the world.*

No additional information changed his mind. A solution to this problem was reached when the patient cheerfully accepted a suggestion that alternating six days on and one day off could comfortably accommodate both the doctor's and the patient's concerns.

This example demonstrates the doctor's ability to *listen* and *respond.* He did not hesitate to step into the patient's world, look at life through his patient's eyes for a moment, and "discover" that *in that world* hypertension medications *were* poison and taking pills for six months and discontinuing them for six months really meant "taking your pills." He also could see that within his patient's perspective one *must* flush out the poison—no questions asked!

This physician then shifted his weight to his theoretical base of *medical knowledge.* He realized that six consistent days of medication would adequately protect his patient and would certainly be better than six months off. He then "balanced his weight," planted both feet firmly, and planned. He proposed an intervention within the context of his patient's model, that was healthier than that developed by the patient.

Nevertheless, later when he reported this incident, this physician described it as a strange and unexpected case. Because he sees the situation this way it is most unlikely that he is systematic, comprehensive, and holistic in his approach.

Q11: What particular needs of persons can be met by nurses practicing independently or collaboratively with physicians from offices or in homes?

It is widely acknowledged that 75% to 80% of those who visit doctors' offices do not need a physician's special expertise. They may be experiencing physical symptoms as a signal of difficulties in their relationships or lifestyle, or they may be using office visits consciously or unconsciously as social and emotional outlets. Visiting physicians over and over without gaining relief, they place themselves in jeopardy of unnecessary tests and medical treatments that waste time and money at best and create iatrogenic problems at worst.

Nurses in private practice have the potential to demonstrate newer and more effective ways of delivering needed health care. If more experienced nurses would make themselves available to the public in private practices, they would significantly help this large group of discouraged and discouraging clients. After making thorough checkups to rule out organic and treatable tissue involvement, physicians could refer those with lingering and vague complaints to nurses for the nursing care they are actually seeking. When a problem relating to life situations and relationships is thought to be causing physical distress symptoms, a nurse is ideally suited to give holistic assistance.

Payment for these services by third parties still needs to be arranged through political and legislative means. Because it is difficult to find ways to prove disease *prevention* as opposed to *early detection*, we may need to argue that such care at the very least will reduce our skyrocketing national expenditures for unnecessary hospitalizations and for many preventable medical–surgical complications.

There will always be people who need a physician's expertise in the diagnosis and treatment of their physical abnormalities, dysfunctions, injuries, burns, infections, tumors, and diseases. Those who need help adhering to prescribed regimes of daily care for these and long-standing chronic disorders could see nurses regularly in offices and homes to help them cope with all the manifestations of their anxiety, whether physical, mental, emotional, social, cultural, or spiritual. Professional nurses alone have the formal preparation and expertise needed to foster in their clients a high level of holistic wellness as their clients continue growing and developing throughout their lives.

Glossary

Accommodation   The establishment of a new schema (framework or structure) or the re-structuring of an old schema (pl. schemata) in order to take in new information.

Adaptation   The process by which an individual responds to external and internal stressors in a health and growth-directed manner.

Adaptation energy   The energy necessary to acquire and maintain adaptation, apart from caloric requirements. (Hans Selye, *The Stress of Life*, p. 463.)

Adaptive equilibrium   State in which people who have a good potential for mobilizing coping resources use them in a growth and health-directed manner that leaves no subsystem in jeopardy.

Affiliated–Individuation   The need to be able to be dependent on support systems while simultaneously maintaining independence from these support systems.

Aggregate   To compile or gather together individual pieces of information.

Analyze   To examine critically so as to bring out the essential elements.

APAM   Abbreviation for *adaptive potential assessment model* which identifies three states of coping: *arousal, equilibrium,* and *impoverishment.* Each state represents a different potential for mobilizing resources needed to contend with stressors.

Arousal   One of the states of the APAM, a stress state.

Assimilation   The cognitive process by which one takes in and integrates new perceptual stimuli into existing schemata or patterns.

Client   One who is considered to be a legitimate member of the decision-making team, who always has some control over the planned regimen, and who is incorporated in his or her own care as much as possible.

Cognitive processes   Mental processes that reflect thinking, reasoning, and problem solving. Cognitive processes exclude affective processes.

Coping   The process of contending with stressors. Coping can be adaptive (health and growth-directed) or maladaptive (sickness-directed).

Development   The holistic synthesis of the growth-produced increasing differentiations of a person's body, ideas, social relations, and so forth.

Distressor   A stimulus that is experienced as threatening or one that mounts (either directly or indirectly) a maladaptive response.

Equilibration   The balance between assimilation and accommodation.

Equilibrium   A state of the APAM, wherein persons have a good potential for mobilizing coping resources.

Facilitation   Making easier or less difficult; helping forward. The nurse–client relationship is an interactive process that helps the individual to identify, mobilize, and develop the individual's own strengths in his or her movement toward health.

Growth   The changes in body, mind, and spirit that occur over time.

Health   A state of physical, mental, and social well-being, not merely the absence of disease or infirmity. Additionally, it connotes a state of equilibrium within each of the various subsystems of a holistic person.

Holism   The concept that a multisystem person is more than the mere sum of subsystem parts and inherent bases; it stresses the dynamic interaction of subsystems and inherent bases.

Impoverishment   A state of the APAM, wherein persons have diminished, if not depleted, resources available for mobilization.

Maladaptation   The process an individual uses to cope with a stressor within one subsystem by taxing energies from another.

Maladaptive equilibrium   A relatively steady state wherein an individual is coping with stressors but at the cost of draining energies from another subsystem or subsystems.

Model   The standard or representation being replicated.

Modeling   The process used by the nurse as she develops an image and understanding of the client's world, as the client perceives it.

Nurturance   The fusing and integrating of cognitive, physiological, and affective processes with the aim of assisting a client to move toward holistic health.

Paradigm   A structure, framework, pattern, or form to guide and direct practice.

Patient   One who is given aid, instruction, and treatment with the expectation that such services are appropriate and that the recipient will accept them and comply with the plan.

Role-modeling   The facilitation and nurturance of the individual in attaining, maintaining or promoting health through purposeful interventions.

Schemata (plural of schema)   The cognitive structural units that continually change in shape by which individuals adapt to and organize their environment intellectually.

Self-care actions   The development and utilization of self-care knowledge and self-care resources.

Self-care knowledge   At some level a person knows what has made him or her sick, lessened his or her effectiveness or interfered with his or her growth. The person also knows what will make him or her well, optimize his or her effectiveness or fulfillment (given the circumstances) or promote his or her growth.

Self-care resources: The internal resources, as well as additional resources, mobilized through self-care action that will help gain, maintain, and promote an optimum level of holistic health.

Stress The nonspecific response of the holistic person to any demand.

Stressor A stimulus that precedes and elicits stress.

Synthesize To integrate into a holistic unit.

Theory A set of systematically presented concepts that explains, relates, predicts, and prescribes specific phenomena.

Unconditional acceptance Being accepted as a unique, worthwhile, important individual with no strings attached. The nurse uses empathy to invite the client into this perception.

Wholism The state in which the whole is equal to the sum of the parts.

Bibliography

CHAPTER ONE

Chaska, N. L. *The Nursing Profession: Views through the Mist.* New York: McGraw-Hill, 1978.

Claus, K. E., and Bailey, J. T. *Power and Influence in Health Care.* Saint Louis: C. V. Mosby Co., 1977.

Goodwin, L., and Taylor, N. "Doing Away with the 'Doctor–Nurse Game'." *Supervisor Nurse* 8 (June 1977): 25–26.

Kalisch, P., and Kalisch, B. "An Analysis of the Sources of Physician–Nurse Conflict." *Journal of Nursing Administration* 7 (Jan. 1977): 51–57.

———. *The Advance of American Nursing.* Boston: Little, Brown and Co., 1978.

Lysaught, J. *Action in Nursing: Progress in Professional Purpose.* New York: McGraw-Hill, 1974.

McGuire, M. "Nurse–Physician Interactions: Silence Isn't Golden." *Supervisor Nurse* 11 (1980): 36–39.

Mallison, M. B. "Our Eyes Are on Results." *American Journal of Nursing* 81 (1981): 1813.

"Nurse–Physician Interactions." Film strip, The University of Michigan Media Library, Ann Arbor, Michigan, 1977.

Pardue, S. F. "Assertiveness for Nursing." *Supervisor Nurse* 11 (Feb. 1980): 47–50.

Pearlmutter, D. "Dissent and Conflict in the Health Professions." In *No Rush to Judgment: Essays on Medical Ethics*, edited by Smith and Bernstein, pp. 221-37. Bloomington: Poynter Center, 1978.

_____ and Warner, G. M. "Attitudes of Physicians to Nurses." *New York State Journal of Medicine* 70 (1970): 2840–46.

Richards, R. "The Game Professionals Play." *Supervisor Nurse* 9 (June 1978): 48–50.

Sheard, T. "The Structure of Conflict in Nurse–Physician Relations." *Supervisor Nurse* 11 (Aug. 1980): 14–18.

Smith, D. R. "What is the Professional Nurse (*Really?*)." *Supervisor Nurse* 11 (May 1980): 34–35.

CHAPTER TWO

Abdellah, F. G.; Beland, I.; Martin, A.; and Matheney, R. *New Directions in Patient-centered Nursing*. New York: Macmillan, 1973.

_____. *Patient-centered Approaches to Nursing*. New York: Macmillan, 1960.

Frederick, H. K., and Northam, E. *A Textbook of Nursing Practice*, 2d ed. New York: Macmillan, 1938.

Harmer, B. *Textbook of the Principles and Practice of Nursing*, 5th ed., rev. V. Henderson. New York: Macmillan, 1955.

Henderson, V. *ICN Basic Principles of Nursing Care*. London: ICN (International Council of Nurses) House, 1960.

_____. *The Nature of Nursing*. New York: Macmillan, 1966.

Johnson, D. E. "The Significance of Nursing Care." *American Journal of Nursing* 61 (Nov. 1961): 63–65.

Joseph, L. "Self-Care and the Nursing Process." *Nursing Clinics of North America* 15 (March 1980): 131–43.

Kaplan, A. *The Conduct of Inquiry*. San Francisco: Chandler, 1964.

King, I. E. *Toward a Theory for Nursing: General Concepts of Human Behavior*. New York: John Wiley, 1971.

Kinlein, M. L. *Independent Nursing Practice With Clients*. Philadelphia: Lippincott, 1977.

Krieger, D. *Therapeutic Touch: How to Use Your Hands to Help and Heal*. Englewood Cliffs, N.J.: Prentice-Hall, 1979.

Levine, M. E. *Introduction to Clinical Nursing*, 2d ed. Philadelphia: Davis, 1973.

Maslow, A. *The Psychology of Science: A Reconnaisance*. New York: Harper & Row, Pub., 1966.

Mitchell, P. H. *Concepts Basic to Nursing*, 2d ed. New York: McGraw-Hill, 1973.

Nightingale, F. *Notes on Nursing: What It Is and What It Is Not*. London: Harrison, 1859, 1914.

――――. "Sick Nursing and Health Nursing." In *Nursing of the Sick*, edited by I. Hampton et al., 1893. New York: McGraw-Hill, 1949.

Nursing Development Conference Group. *Concept Formalization in Nursing: Process and Product*. Boston: Little, Brown and Co., 1973.

Orem, D. E. *Nursing: Concepts of Practice*. New York: McGraw-Hill, 1971.

Orlando, I. J. *The Discipline and Teaching of Nursing Process: (An Evaluative Study)*. New York: Putnam's, 1972.

――――. *The Dynamic Nurse–Patient Relationship*. New York: Putnam's, 1961.

Peplau, H. E. *Interpersonal Relations in Nursing: A Conceptual Frame of Reference for Psychodynamic Nursing*. New York: Putnam's, 1952.

Riehl, J., and Roy, C. *Conceptual Models for Nursing Practice*. New York: Appleton-Century-Crofts, 1974.

Rogers, M. *Educational Revolution in Nursing*. New York: Macmillan, 1961.

――――. *An Introduction to the Theoretical Basis of Nursing*. Philadelphia: Davis, 1970.

Roy, C. *Introduction to Nursing: An Adaptation Model*. Englewood Cliffs, N.J.: Prentice-Hall, 1976.

Shaw, C. S. W. *A Textbook of Nursing.* New York: Appleton, 1885, 1902.

Travelbee, J. *Interpersonal Aspects of Nursing.* Philadelphia: Davis, 1966.

————. *Interpersonal Aspects of Nursing,* 2d ed. Philadelphia: Davis, 1971.

Wiedenbach, E. *Clinical Nursing: A Helping Art.* New York: Springer, 1964.

————. "Nurses' Wisdom in Nursing Theory." *American Journal of Nursing* 70 (1970): 1057-62.

CHAPTER THREE

Banham, K. "The Development of Affectionate Behavior in Infancy." In *Human Development,* 2d ed., eds. M. Haimowitz and N. Haimowitz, pp. 206-12. New York: Thomas Y. Crowell, 1960.

Flynn, P. *Holistic Health: The Art and Science of Care.* Bowie, Md.: Brady, 1981.

Levy, D. M. "Maternal Overprotection." In *Human Development,* 2d ed., edited by M. Haimowitz and N. Haimowitz, pp. 399-407.

CHAPTER FOUR

Anderson, C. "Aspects of Pathological Grief and Mourning." *International Journal of Psychoanalysis* 30 (1949): 48-55.

Arthur, B., and Kemme, M. "Bereavement in Childhood." *Journal of Child Psychology and Psychiatry* 5 (1964): 37-49.

Barry, H. "The Significance of Maternal Bereavement before Age Eight in Psychotic Patients." *Archives of Neurology and Psychiatry* 62 (1949): 630-37.

————, and Lindemann, E. "Critical Ages for Bereavement in Psychoneurosis." *Psychosomatic Medicine* 22 (1960): 166-81.

Bartrop, R. W.; Lazarus, L.; Luckhurst, E.; Kiloh, L. G.; and Penny, R. "Depressed Lymphocyte Function After Bereavement." *The Lancet* 1 (1977): 834-36.

Bowlby, J. *Attachment.* New York: Basic Books, 1969.

————. "Child Care and the Growth of Love." In *Human Develop-ment,* 2d ed., edited by M. Haimowitz and N. Haimowitz, pp. 155–66. New York: Thomas Y. Crowell, 1960.

————. "Childhood Mourning and Its Explications for Psychiatry." *American Journal of Psychiatry* 118 (1961): 481–98.

————. *Loss.* New York: Basic Books, 1980.

————. "The Nature of the Child's Tie to His Mother," *International Journal of Psychoanalysis* 39 (1958): 89–97.

————. "Process of Mourning." *International Journal of Psycho-analysis* 42 (1961): 317–40.

————. *Separation.* New York: Basic Books, 1973.

————, Robertson, J.; and Rosenbluth, D. "A Two-Year-Old Goes to the Hospital." *The Psychoanalytic Study of the Child* 7 (1952): 89–94.

Brody, S. "Transitional Objects: Idealization of a Phenomenon." *Psychoanalytic Quarterly* 49 (1980): 561–601.

Brown, F. "Depression and Childhood Bereavement." *Journal of Mental Science* 107 (1961): 754–77.

Cassel, J. "The Contribution of the Social Environment to Host Re-sistance." *American Journal of Epidemiology* 104 (1976): 107–23.

Deutsch, H. "The Absence of Grief." *Psychoanalytic Quarterly* 6 (1937): 12–22.

Dohrenwend, B. "Life Events as Stressors: A Methodological In-quiry." *Journal of Health and Social Behavior* 14 (1973): 167–75.

Donahue, P. "Concepts of Loss and Grief." In *The Process of Hu-man Development: A Holistic Approach,* edited by C. Schuster and L. Ashburn, pp. 785–796. Boston: Little, Brown and Co., 1980.

Drake, R., and Price, J. L. "Depression: Adaptation to Disruption and Loss." *Perspectives in Psychiatric Care* 13 (1975): 163–69.

Engel, G. S. *Psychological Development in Health and Disease.* Philadelphia: Saunders, 1962.

Erikson, E. *Childhood and Society.* New York: W. W. Norton & Co., Inc., 1963.

————. "Identity Versus Self-Diffusion." In *Human Development,* 2d ed., edited by M. Haimowitz and N. Haimowitz, pp. 766–70.

Flynn, P. *Holistic Health: The Art and Science of Care*. Bowie, Md.: Brady, 1981.

Fraiberg, S. "The Origin of Human Bonds." *Commentary* 44 (1967): 47–57.

Freedman, A. M.; Kaplan, H. I.; and Sadock, B. J. *Modern Synopsis of Comprehensive Textbook of Psychotherapy II*. Baltimore: Williams & Wilkins, 1976.

Gable, F. *The Third Force*. New York: Pocket Books, 1974.

Glass, D. "Stress, Behavior Patterns, and Coronary Disease." *American Scientist* 65 (1977): 177–87.

Haimowitz, M. L. "Criminals Are Made, Not Born." In *Human Development*, 2d ed., edited by M. Haimowitz and N. Haimowitz, pp. 359–375.

Harlan, W. "Physical and Psychosocial Stress and the Cardiovascular System." (AHA Task Force Report) *Circulation* 63 (1981): 266-A–271-A.

Harlow, H. "The Nature of Love." In *Human Development*, 2d ed., edited by M. Haimowitz and N. Haimowitz, pp. 190–206.

Hinkle, L. E. "The Effect of Exposure to Culture Change, Social Change, and Changes in Interpersonal Relationships on Health." In *Stressful Life Events: Their Nature and Effects*, edited by B. S. Dohrenwend and B. P. Dohrenwend, pp. 9–44. New York: John Wiley, 1974.

———, and Wolf, S. "A Summary of Experimental Evidence Relating Life Stress to Diabetes Mellitus." *Mt. Sinai Journal of Medicine in New York* 19 (1952): 537–570.

Holmes, T. H., and Masuda, M. "Life change and illness susceptibility." In *Stressful Life Events: Their Nature and Effects*, edited by B. S. Dohrenwend and B. P. Dohrenwend, pp. 45–72. New York: John Wiley, 1974.

———, and Rahe, R. H. "The Social Readjustment Rating Scale." *Journal of Psychosomatic Research* 11 (1967): 213–218.

Hurst, M. W.; Jenkins, C. D.; and Rose, R. M. "The Relation of Psychological Stress to Onset of Medical Illness." In *Stress and Survival*, edited by C. Garfield, pp. 17–26. St. Louis: C. V. Mosby. 1979.

Kimball, C. P. "Conceptual Development in Psychosomatic Medicine: 1939–1969." *Annals of Internal Medicine* 73 (1970): 307–16.

Klein, M. "Some Theoretical Conclusions Regarding the Emotional Life of the Infant." In *Developments in Psycho-Analysis,* edited by J. Riviere, pp. 198–236. London: Hogarth Press, 1952.

Lindemann, E. "Symptomatology and Management of Acute Grief." *American Journal of Psychiatry* 101 (1944): 141–48.

Mahler, M. S. "On Human Symbiosis and the Vicissitudes of Individuation." *J. Amer. Psa. Assn.* 15 (1967): pp. 740–763.

—— and Furer, M. *On Human Symbiosis and the Vicissitudes of Individuation. Vol. I. Infantile Psychosis.* New York: International Universities Press, Inc., 1968.

Maslow, A. H. *Motivation and Personality,* 2d ed. New York: Harper & Row, Pub., 1970.

——. "The Need to Know and the Fear of Knowing." *The Journal of General Psychology* 68 (1936): 111–25.

——. *Toward a Psychology of Being,* 2d ed. New York: D. Van Nostrand, 1968.

Miller, C.; Stein, R.; and Grim, C. "Personality Factors of the Hypertensive Patient." *International Journal of Nursing Studies* 16 (1979): 235–51.

Miller, H., and Baruch, D. W. "A Study of Hostility in Allergic Children." In *Human Development,* 2d ed., edited by M. Haimowitz and N. Haimowitz, pp. 432–43.

Murray, R., and Zentner, J. *Nursing Concepts for Health Promotion,* 2nd ed. Englewood Cliffs, N.J.: Prentice-Hall, 1979.

Pelletier, K. *Mind as Healer, Mind as Slayer.* New York: Delta, 1977.

Piaget, J., and Inhelder, B. *The Psychology of the Child.* New York: Basic Books, 1969.

——. "The Pathway between Subjects' Recent Life Changes and Their Near-Future Illness Reports: Representative Results and Methodological Issues." In *Stressful Life Events: Their Nature and Effects,* edited by B. S. Dohrenwend and B. P. Dohrenwend, pp. 73–86. New York: John Wiley, 1974.

Rahe, R. H., and Arthur, R. J. "Life Change and Illness Studies: Past History and Future Directions." *Journal of Human Stress* 4 (1978): 3–15.

Redl, F. "Children Who Hate." In *Human Development,* 2d ed., edited by M. Haimowitz and N. Haimowitz, pp. 375–90.

Rochlin, G. "The Dread of Abandonment. A Contribution to the Etiology of the Loss Complex and to Depression." *The Psychoanalytic Study of the Child* 16 (1961): 451–70.

Schuster, C. S., and Ashburn, S. S. *The Process of Human Development: A Holistic Approach*. Boston: Little, Brown and Co., 1980.

Seligman, M. "Helplessness." In *The Psychology of Depression: Contemporary Theory and Research*, vol. 2, edited by R. J. Friedman and M. M. Katz, pp. 83–125. Washington, D.C.: V. H. Winston and Sons, 1974.

Spitz, R. "Motherless Infants." In *Human Development*, 2d ed. edited by M. Haimowitz and N. Haimowitz, pp. 166–173.

Volicer, B. "Hospital Stress and Patient Reports of Pain and Physical Status." *Journal of Human Stress* 4 (1978): 28–37.

Winnicott, D. W. "The Theory of the Parent-Infant Relationship. In *The Maturational Processes and the Facilitating Environment*, pp. 37–55. London: The Hogarth Press, 1965.

———. "Transitional Objects and Transitional Phenomena. A Study of the First Not-Me Possession." *Int. J. Psa.* 34 (1953): 89–97.

Wolff, H. G. "Life Stress and Bodily Disease—a Formulation." In *Life Stress and Bodily Disease*, edited by H. G. Wolff, S. G. Wolf, & C. C. Hare, pp. 1059–1094. Baltimore: The Williams and Wilkins Company, 1950.

CHAPTER FIVE

Aakster, C. W. "Psycho-social Stress and Health Disturbances." *Social Science and Medicine* 8 (1974): 77–90.

Arce, L. "Somatopsychic Disease." *Psychosomatics* 13 (1972): 191–96.

Cooper, G. *The Stress Check. Coping with the Stress of Life and Work*. Englewood Cliffs, N.J.: Prentice-Hall, Spectrum Books, 1981.

Garfield, C., ed., *Stress and Survival*. St. Louis: C. V. Mosby, 1980.

Goldstein, A. M. "The Subjective Experience of Denial in an Objective Investigation of Chronically Ill Patients." *Psychosomatics* 13 (1972): 20–22.

Gordon, David, and Anderson, Maribeth. *Phoenix* (Cupertino, California: Meta Publications, 1981).

Laborit, H. "On the Mechanism of Activation of the Hypothalmo-pituitary-adrenal Reaction to Changes in the Environment (The Alarm Reaction)." *Resuscitation* 5 (1976): 19–30.

Lamb, D. H. "On the Distinction between Psychological and Physical Stressors." *Psychological Reports* 38 (1976): 797–98.

Lambert, V., and Lambert, C. *The Impact and Physical Illness and Related Mental Health Concepts.* Englewood Cliffs, N.J.: Prentice-Hall, 1979.

Llorens, L. A. "The Effects of Stress on Growth and Development." *American Journal of Occupational Therapists* 28 (1974): 82–86.

Mills, I. H. "The Disease of Failure of Coping." *Practitioner* 217 (1976): 529–38.

Moss, M. "Heart Under Seige: New Stress on Stress." *Emergency Medicine* 9 (Sept. 1977): 35–51.

Seligman, M. *Helplessness.* San Francisco: W. H. Freeman & Company, Publishers, 1975.

Selye, H. "Further Thoughts on Stress Without Distress." *Resident and Staff Physican* 25 (1979): 125–34.

———. *The Stress of Life*, 2d ed. New York: McGraw-Hill, 1976.

———. *Stress Without Distress.* Philadelphia: Lippincott, 1974.

Shmagin, B., and Pearlmutter, D. "The Pursuit of Unhappiness: The Secondary Gains of Depression." *Perspectives of Psychiatric Care* 15, or Vol. 15, no. 2 (1977): 63–65.

Volicer, B. J. "Hospital Stress and Patient Reports of Pain and Physical Status." *Journal of Human Stress* 4 (June 1978): 28–37.

CHAPTER SIX

Fraiberg, S. "Libidinal Object Constancy and Mental Representation." *The Psychoanalytical Study of the Child* 24 (1969): 9–47.

———. *The Magic Years.* New York: Scribners', 1959.

Luparello, T. "Chronic Illness, Conflict and the Self: Part I—For Some Illness Pays." *Medical Insight* 6 (Jan. 1974): 24–30.

_____. "Chronic Illness, Conflict and the Self: Part II—For Some Illness Pays." *Medical Insight* 6 (Feb. 1974): 12-19.

Robertson, J., and Robertson, J. "Quality of Substitute Care as an Influence on Separation Responses." *Journal of Psychosomatic Research* 16 (1972): 261-65.

Sander, L. "Issues in Early Mother-Child Interaction." *Journal of the American Academy of Child Psychiatry* 1 (1962): 141-67.

CHAPTER SEVEN

Becker, M. H.; Drachman, R. H.; and Kirscht, J. P. "Motivations as Predictors of Health Behavior." *Health Services Report* 87 (1972): 852-62.

Becker, M. H.; Rodius, S. M.; Rosenstock, I. M.; Drachman, R. N.; Schuberth, K. C.; and Teets, K. C. "Compliance with a Medical Regimen for Asthma: A Test of the Health Belief Model." *Public Health Reports* 93 (1978): 268-77.

Blackwell, B. "Patient Compliance." *New England Journal of Medicine* 289 (1973): 249-52.

Boyd, J. and others. "Drug Defaulting Part I: Determinants of Compliance." *American Journal of Hospital Pharmacy* 31 (1974): 362-67.

Cummings, K. M.; Jette, A. M.; and Rosenstock, I. M. "Constant Validation of the Health Belief Model." *Health Education Monographs*, 1979.

Erikson, E. "The Case of Peter." In *Human Development*, edited by M. Haimowitz and N. Haimowitz, 2d ed., pp. 355-359. New York: Thomas Y. Crowell, 1960.

Georgopoulos, B. S., and Mann, F. "The Hospital as an Organization." In *Patients, Physicians and Illness*, 2d ed., edited by E. G. Jaco, pp. 296-305. New York: Free Press, 1972.

Gillium, R. F., and Barsky, A. J. "Diagnosis and Management of Patient Noncompliance." *Journal of the American Medical Association* 228 (1974): 1563-67.

Gladstone, T., and McKegney, F. P. "Relationship Between Patient Behaviors and Nursing Staff Attitudes." *Supervisor Nurse* 11 (1980): 32-35.

Haynes, R. B.; Sackett, D. L.; and Taylor, D. W. "How to Detect and Manage Low Patient Compliance in Chronic Illness." *Geriatrics* 35 (1980): 91–99.

Hingson, R. W. "The Physician's Problems in Identifying Potentially Non-compliant Patients." In *Medication Compliance: A Behavioral Management Approach*, edited by I. Barofsky, pp. 117–132. Thorofare, N.J.; Charles B. Slack, 1977.

Kleinman, A. M. "Exploratory Models in Health Care Relationships." Monograph for *International Health Conference on Health of the Family*. Washington, D.C.: National Council for International Health, 1974.

Lowe, K., and Kutzker, J. "Increasing Compliance to a Medical Regimen with a Juvenile Diabetic." *Behavior Therapy* 10 (1979): 57–64.

Marston, M. "Compliance with Medical Regimes: A Review of the Literature." *Nursing Research* 19 (1970): 312–23.

Polanyi, M. *Personal Knowledge: Towards a Post-Critical Philosophy*. Chicago: University of Chicago Press, 1962.

Rosenstock, I. M. "Why People use Health Services." *Milbank Memorial Fund Quarterly* 44 (1966): 94–124.

Sackett, D. L., and Haynes, R. B., eds. *Compliance with Therapeutic Regimens*. Baltimore: Johns Hopkins University Press, 1976.

Sackett, D. L., and Snow, J. "The Magnitude of Compliance and Noncompliance." In *Compliance in Health Care*, edited by R. B. Haynes, D. W. Taylor, and D. L. Sackett, pp. 475–507. Baltimore: Johns Hopkins University Press, 1979.

Williamson, J. "Mutual Interaction: A Model of Nursing Practice." *Nursing Outlook* 29 (1981): 104–07.

Wu, R. *Behavior and Illness*. Englewood Cliffs, N.J.: Prentice-Hall, 1973.

CHAPTER EIGHT

Becker, M. H. *The Health Belief Model and Personal Health Behavior*. Thorofare, N.J.: Charles B. Slack, 1974.

Jaco, E. G., ed. *Patients, Physicians, and Illiness: A Sourcebook in Behavioral Science and Health*, 3d ed. New York: Free Press, 1979.

Jasmin, S., and Trygstad, L. N. *Behavioral Concepts and the Nursing Process*. Saint Louis: C. V. Mosby, 1979.

CHAPTER NINE

Carpenter, S. "Family-Focused Interventions." In *Mental Health Concepts Applied to Nursing*, edited by N. L. Dunlap, pp. 128–135. New York: John Wiley, 1978.

Lindemann, E. "Symptomatology and Management of Acute Grief." *American Journal of Psychiatry* 101 (1944): 141–148.

Nierenberg, G. J., and Calero, H. H. *How to Read a Person Like a Book*. New York: Pocket Books, 1975.

CHAPTER TEN

Lambert, V. A., and Lambert, C. E. *The Impact of Physical Illness and Related Mental Health Concepts*. Englewood Cliffs, N.J.: Prentice-Hall, 1979.

Roberts, S. *Behavioral Concepts and Nursing Throughout the Life Span*. Englewood Cliffs, N.J.: Prentice-Hall, 1978.

CHAPTER ELEVEN

Benjamin, A. *The Helping Interview*, 2d ed. Boston: Houghton-Mifflin Company, 1969.

Brill, N. I. *Working with People: The Helping Process*. Philadelphia: J. B. Lippincott Company, 1973.

Carlsmith, J. B., Collins, B. E., and Helmreide, R. L. "Studies in Forced Compliance." *Journal of Personality and Social Psychology* 4 (1966): 1–13.

Centi, Paul. *Up with the Positive, Out With the Negative: How to Like the Person You Are.* Englewood Cliffs, N.J.: Prentice-Hall, Inc. (A Spectrum Book), 1981.

Chapman, J. S. "Effects of Different Nursing Approaches on Psychological and Physiological Responses," *Nursing Research Report* 5 (March 1970): 5-7.

Claus, K. E., and Bailey, J. T. *Living With Stress and Promoting Well-Being.* St. Louis: C. V. Mosby Co., 1980.

Erickson, H. "Communications in Nursing." In *Professional Nursing Matrix: A Workbook*, pp. I-3-I-189. The University of Michigan Media Library, Ann Arbor, Michigan, 1977.

Fertig, R. D. "Reaching Rejected Youth." In *Human Development*, edited by M. Haimowitz and N. Haimowitz, 2d ed., pp. 616-27. New York: Thomas Crowell Co., 1960.

Foster, S. "An Adrenal Measure For Evaluating Nursing Effectiveness." *Nursing Research*, 23 (1974): 118-22.

Frankenhaeuser, M. "Experimental Approaches to the Study of Catecholamines and Emotions." In *Emotions: Their Parameters and Measurements*, edited by L. Levi, pp. 209-234. New York: Raven Press, 1975.

Ginott, H. G. *Between Parent and Child.* New York: Avon Books, 1965.

Harris, S. J. *Winners and Losers.* Allen, Texas: Argus Communications, 1973.

Highriter, M. E. "Nurse Characteristics and Patient Progress." *Nursing Research* 18 (1969): 484-92.

Jourard, S. "Suicide. An Invitation to Die." *American Journal of Nursing* 70 (1970): 269-75.

Knapp, T. J., and Peterson, L. W. "Behavior Management in Medical and Nursing Practice." In *Application of Behavior Modification: Principles, Issues and Applications*, edited by N. E. Craighead et al., pp. 260-288. Boston: Houghton-Mifflin, 1976.

Langer, E. G., and Rodin, J. "The Effects of Choice and Enhanced Personal Responsibility for the Aged: A Field Experiment in an Institutional Setting." *Journal of Personality and Social Psychology* 34 (1976): 191-98.

MacMillan, P. "Spacing and Touching and Hugging." *Nursing Times* 77 (April 30, 1981): 788-90.

James, M., and Jongeward, D. *Born to Win*. Reading, Mass.: Addison-Wesley, 1971.

Nightingale, F. *Notes on Nursing: What It Is and What It Is Not*. New York: D. Appleton, 1860.

Northouse, P. "Interpersonal Trust and Empathy in Nurse–Nurse Relationships." *Nursing Research* 28 (1979): 365–68.

Rogers, C., and Stevens, B. *Person to Person: The Problem of Being Human*. New York: Pocket Books, 1967.

Satir, V. *Making Contact*. Millbrae, Calif.: Celestial Arts, 1976.

Seeman, M. "Patients Who Abandon Psychotherapy: Why and When." *Archives of General Psychiatry* 30 (1974): 486–91.

Selye, H. "Stress Without Distress." In *Stress and Survival*, edited by C. Garfield. St. Louis: C. V. Mosby, 1974.

————. *Stress Without Distress*. Philadelphia: Lippincott, 1974.

Simonton, O.; Simonton, S.; and Creighton, J. *Getting Well Again: A Step-by-Step, Self-Help Guide to Overcoming Cancer for Patients and their Families*. Los Angeles: J. P. Tarcher, Inc., 1978.

Steckel, S. *Patient Contracting*. Englewood Cliffs, N.J.: Prentice-Hall, 1982.

Swain, M. A., and Steckel, S. B. "Influencing Adherence Among Hypertensives." *Research in Nursing and Health* 4 (1981): 213–22.

Talkington, D. R. "Maximizing Patient Compliance by Shaping Attitudes of Self-Directed Health Care." *Journal of Family Practice* 6 (1978): 591–95.

CHAPTER TWELVE

Harris, J. S. *I'm Ok—You're Ok*. New York: Avon Books, 1969.

Lindell, A. "Congruence: A Necessary Behavior of the Nurse–Patient Relationship." *Issues in Mental Health Nursing* 11 (1980): 28–38.

Maltz, M. *The Search for Self Respect*. New York: Bantam Books, 1976.

McNally, J. M. "Values: Part I." *Supervisor Nurse* 11 (1980): 27–29.

———. "Values: Part II." 11 (June 1980): 52–53.

———. "Values: Part III." 11 (July 1980): 17–18.

———. "Values: Part IV." 11 (Aug. 1980): 38–39.

List of the Lengthier Illustrations from Nursing Practice

Index